Following the Drum

Dedication

To Charlie

Preface

As the plane touched down at Nicosia airport a blast of warm air enveloped me. This was the beginning of a whole new adventure. Newly married, newly qualified as a nurse, a whole new set of experiences awaited me. In this, the sequel to Three Years in Starch I am attempting to condense the next 20 to 30 years into 10 chapters.

Chapter 1

The Cyprus Years

As the taxi sped through the small crowded towns, their houses and buildings all leaning in on each other the land gradually gave way to stark barren landscape. Parched from the sun, the yellow grass and stunted trees painted a moonscape type of picture. Here and there a shepherd with a herd of thin sheep ambled along. We passed donkeys laden with what looked like household supplies, blankets and tin kettles, all led by men and women dressed in traditional Greek costume. The men in baggy trousers that ended just below the knee and the women, mainly in black with their heads covered. The Mercedes taxi had no air conditioning and as I had not yet grown acclimatised, the heat was oppressive.

After about an hours driving the taxi stopped. A lone building stood out among the barren landscape. A Union Jack was flying bravely from a flagpole. This was Halfway House, apparently the mid point between Nicosia and Limassol where we would eventually find a house. An ice cold coca cola was welcome after the cramped drive and we sat at one of the small formica covered tables. Within minutes I was surrounded by flies, more flies than I had ever seen in my life. Naturally, I was frantically swatting them away. I noticed my husband and the taxi driver exchange amused looks. "You'll soon get used to them," my husband remarked. I was not convinced. It was bad enough that I had come from a cold and foggy England in November to be greeted by temperatures in excess of 30 degrees, but flies! What else would I be greeted with? After about another hour or so of much the same scenery we approached the outskirts of Limassol. It appeared to be more spacious than Nicosia and there were quite modern looking shops along the route. I have always thought that towns have personalities and Limassol had a nice feel to it. By this time all I wanted was a cool shower. My husband had already done a tour of duty in Libya and had spent two years in Cyprus so he was an old hand, used to the heat and the flies.

We arrived at the hotel where we were to spend two or three days while accommodation was arranged for us. There was no air conditioning, after all, this was

1963, but the ceiling fan moved the air around. After a superb supper of Greek style food, grilled lamb with aubergines and courgettes accompanied by lashings of tangy Greek yoghurt and copious amounts of local red wine I was beginning to think that maybe this wasn't so bad. The next morning while John went to his new unit to sign in and arrange housing I was left to my own devices. The hotel swimming pool provided a welcome diversion and the hotel staff couldn't have been more friendly.

****

House hunting: The next few days were spent in viewing a bizarre selection of Cypriot houses. They ranged from one bedroomed shacks that looked as if the builders had abandoned them half way through, to more opulent three to four bedroom properties with large gardens filled with red geraniums - everywhere were there red geraniums! Growing wild, in window boxes and planted around fences. I learned later the soil was fertile and almost everything grew. Our estate agent, the young Cypriot who was detailed to show us around was a flamboyant character. He would whizz around from house to house in his beat up car at about

60 miles per hour with me gripping the back of the seat as if my life depended on it. He was so enthusiastic about every house he showed us and appeared to take it personally if we declined anything. His expression would change to one of acute distress and I fully expected him to burst into tears. In the end I was tempted to accept anything so as not to hurt his feelings. Fortunately, John, my husband was wise to Cypriot sales tactics.

A strange thing that puzzled me was the fact that many of the houses had reinforced concrete poles sticking out of the roofs. When I remarked on this, Panos, the estate agent told me that it was customary in Cyprus for a father to provide his daughters with a dowry, and this often came in the shape of a house. As many Cypriot families would find it difficult to afford a house outright, they tended to build it in instalments, thus leaving scope for another one or two storeys when they had saved some more money. This explained some of the one bedroomed shacks that I had seen previously.

After two days in which we saw about twenty properties, we finally decided on a pleasant two bedroomed house on the edge of Limassol. It was owned by Sofoulla, a young Greek girl. She was in her 20's, about the same age as me at the time. When I got to know her a bit better she told me the house was her dowry but she would lend it to us until she found a husband. As there appeared to be no handsome young Cypriot on the horizon we hoped that we would be able to occupy it for a while. As with many of the other houses, the upper storey was still waiting to be added.

Then began the process of settling in to the expatriate environment. It was a mixed community of English military and local Cypriots. There was a small shop cum bar a few doors away run by Louis, a middle aged portly Greek. The shop stocked everything you could ask for and if there was something he didn't have it would be there by the next day. I soon grew used to Cyprus bread, the large round loaves fresh out of the oven and halloumi cheese, large white chunks of goats cheese, delicious when served with big red watermelons. It was impossible to go to Louis' shop without being offered a cold coca cola or whatever else the locals were drinking at the time. Cypriot hospitality is legendary and it is thought rude to refuse. The alcohol laws were so lax as to be non existent, and the shelves were stocked with rough red wine and local brandy. At any time of the day I would see three or four of the local men sitting outside the shop drinking bitter coffee and brandy. I would pop over for a loaf of bread and Louis would be effusive in his welcome. "Come, sit, Mrs John," he would say, pulling out a chair. Then he would take a tumbler from the shelf and half fill it with the local brew and maybe a teaspoon of lemonade. I was totally unused to drinking anything stronger than cider in the student bars of Bristol and consequently spent several afternoons flat out asleep on my sofa or nursing a hangover. I suppose my liver adjusted eventually.

Our next door neighbour was Maroulla, and her cat was a thief. His name was Moussa (Moses). I came into the kitchen one day to find him making off with a chicken that I was just about to put into the oven. Maroulla had two sons, Aggie - short for Antonaggi, I think it meant little Aggie, and Bambo. I never did discover whether this was a nickname. They were both about three to five years old, they were both intensely curious about 'Missy John,' and would come and look in my window for hours. They would look away shyly if I tried to speak to them and would never come over the threshold.

As I had not long qualified as a nurse I soon began to think about getting a job. There were several openings for service wives on the army camp, and the medical centre was situated in the town. However, as events transpired it wasn't to be. At least until several years later on our second tour of Cyprus. We had been in the house for about four months when I discovered I was pregnant. Naturally, we were thrilled and Sofoulla was delighted that there would be a baby in her house. It was about this time that the EOKA unrest began to gather pace and the conflict between the Greek and the Turkish side of the Island began to rumble. Around two o clock one morning we were awakened by a massive explosion. It sounded just outside our door and John and I rushed outside to see what had happened. There was a pall of smoke from the direction of Louis' shop and flames lit up the sky. Louis wife - Mrs Louis - was sitting on the grass with her head in her hands and the local women were crowding around her, wailing. Louis himself however, appeared exhilarated. It was the most exciting thing that had happened in years. When I commiserated with him the following morning all he said was. "It's mud and bricks, Mrs John, I will rebuild it." All the villagers rallied round and though we did our shopping from a corrugated iron shed for a few months the shop was eventually rebuilt better than before. It was rumoured around the village that Louis had some connection with the local underground, but rumours were as numerous as the flies in Cyprus.

Sofoulla was a frequent visitor to our house and she loved to tend the garden. This was no problem for me as the temperature was in the 30's and I was in an advanced state of pregnancy. There was a large eucalyptus tree just outside the house and as I was relaxing in its shade I noticed a dead piece of wood sticking out of the ground. I picked it up and threw it on the compost pile. Looking out of the window the next morning I noticed Sofoulla wandering around with a puzzled expression. "Mrs John, Mrs John, where is the grapevine?" she asked. "We don't have a grapevine," I replied, equally puzzled. "I planted one for you yesterday." Light slowly dawned! What was that piece of wood in the compost pile? Yes, that was the new vine that would eventually grow to cover the whole wall. Looking a bit sheepish I retrieved it and we both replanted it. When it grew big and flourished it was forever after known as 'Sophie's vine.'

There were large numbers of stray dogs roaming around on the outskirts of the village and occasionally the 'dog van,' would come and round them up. It was while I was strolling down to the shops I noticed a scruffy mangy looking hound. He looked half starved so I shared my kebab with him. At that moment the dog van came round the corner. The man had what looked like a big fishing net ready to snare any stray dogs. He glanced at the dog, then at me. "Is this your dog, Ma'am?" he enquired. I had a quick think. Not wanting this poor mutt to be taken away to be put in the dog pound or worse, I replied quickly. "Yes, he's mine." The man looked at me dubiously but shrugged and drove on. I hoped that eventually that poor dog found a home.

Another family in the next street had a bitch that was continually having puppies. She had produced three litters in the short time that we had been in the house. They were adorable fluffy little things, and of course, I had to have one. I got out my Greek phrase book and looked up, 'can I buy one of your puppies.' Rehearsing this several times to get the pronunciation right, I marched purposefully over to the house. Hesitantly, I knocked on the door. It was answered by one of the daughters. With a beaming smile she invited me in. "Sit, missy, sit," and the bottle of Cyprus brandy was produced although it was only 10am. The head of the house was summoned together with his wife, and after much small talk in pigeon English, I eventually came to the purpose of my visit. In my best textbook Greek I repeated the phrase I had learned from my book. They all fell about laughing. The daughter, seeing my discomfiture, helped me out. "I think missy John wants a puppy." She said. I agreed eagerly, thankful that at least someone understood me. "Come, come," the daughter said, grabbing my arm, and I was led through the kitchen to the back yard. There, on a blanket was the proud looking bitch with four sandy brown puppies. "Take two," said the man. "They are fine puppies, Yes." I replied that one would be fine, and I was quite happy to buy it. The man opened his mouth to say I could have the puppy for nothing, but the Mama, obviously the business brains of the family, cut in before he could continue. "Five Cyprus pounds missy John." I was quite happy with the price, as I had been prepared to pay twice that amount. I had not yet learned that they expected me to bargain. So I acquired Benjy, a lovely boisterous Cyprus hound. He became my constant companion but I could never teach him any tricks. Frankly, he was a bit dim. He would eat anything, and once when I dropped a packet of lard on the kitchen floor he had devoured it before I could reach for a cloth to pick it up. Who needs a hoover when you have a puppy?

Somehow word had got around to the local community that I was a trained nurse, and occasionally there would be a knock at the door and a mother would appear with a child with a cut head or finger. I would patch them up and the next day a large bunch of grapes or a basket of luscious Greek tomatoes would appear on my doorstep.

Although life in Limassol appeared idyllic and peaceful there was much tension bubbling under the surface. EOKA, the underground Greek Cypriot organisation regarded as terrorists, wanted union with Greece. The Turkish Cypriots disagreed. EOKA was carrying out a campaign of bombings and unrest mainly against the British military up until 1960 when Cyprus was granted independence from Britain, with the exception of two SBA's (sovereign base areas) which Britain kept on as strategic bases. Back in the 1950's Ledra Street in Nicosia - the infamous 'murder mile,' was where much of the fighting took place. Occasionally the unrest would bubble over and the situation would be classed as an alert. These alerts followed a colour code ranging from green to red, green being low risk of attack, through blue, yellow, orange and red. Red, of course, being a serious or imminent risk.

As a young wife living in what I regarded as the relative safety of the military family community in Limassol I was quite unprepared for what followed. I had grown used to the sound of gunfire, indeed it had been going on sporadically for some weeks. It was 2am when there was a frantic knocking on our door. A close friend and his wife were living a few miles away in the Turkish quarter when there was a flare up of hostilities. Apparently Jane, the wife had spent the previous evening and night under the table in their kitchen as bombs rocked the house and bullets whistled over her head. When there was a lull in the fighting Bob, the husband grabbed his wife and baby, and jumping in his beat up old car, made a dash for anywhere that was relatively safe, in this case, it was our house. When morning came they were escorted by the military back to their house to retrieve some of their clothes and baby food. It was an incongruous sight. At the head of the convoy was a large Armoured Vehicle, then our tiny Fiat 500 followed by Bob's small car and another massive Armoured vehicle bringing up the rear. They stayed with us for three days then arrangements were made to rehouse them.

All this time the British newspapers were running lurid stories about the unrest in Cyprus and there were frequent references to Limassol and Nicosia. My father, back home in Wales must have been extremely worried especially as there was no telephone link or mobile phones as there are today. The worst actual fighting I ever saw was a group of young Greek Cypriots with guns. They would spring out from behind a tree or round a corner, fire shots into the air and dash back to where they had come from. I imagine a lot of ammunition was discharged in that way. Not to say that the fighting wasn't serious in many other areas. Horror stories are told to this day, and with good reason.

About this time my puppy, Benjy, became ill. I caught him trying to eat a dead bird, feathers and all. I was unable to retrieve it before he wolfed it down. The following day he didn't rush to greet me, he just lay in his basket. By the evening it was obvious that something was terribly wrong. It was a Saturday and the nearest vet was closed. Poor old Benjy wouldn't even take sips of water and I sat up all night. In the early hours of the morning he stirred, licked my hand and fell back. Gradually I watched him stop breathing. With tears rolling down my cheeks I got my husband out of bed. As I cried on his shoulder suddenly all the windows in the house shook and rattled. This was much more than the usual, 'play fighting,' as we had come to regard it. The village church had received a direct hit and the shelling continued for the rest of the day. We realised that if this went on much longer we would have to pack a few belongings and allow the military to evacuate us on to the base. I wasn't going to leave Benjy to the scavengers and I insisted on burying him decently. A prized possession, the laundry bag that had accompanied me all through my nurses training was unearthed from a box in the spare room. With much reverence Benjy was wrapped in it while we dug a deep hole in the garden. The bombing continued although it had moved away from our direct area. Benjy was buried and I planted geraniums all around the patch. Later that day we learned that we were on Red Alert and we were advised to keep 24 hours supply of food in the house for the foreseeable future. Also we were to be prepared to move at a moment's notice if necessary.

As the noise and fighting abated, my pregnancy progressed. It was mid June with temperatures soaring to 32 degrees when Jimmy arrived. My first born and my dad's first grandchild. The new hospital in Akrotiri, the neighbouring sovereign base area had been open for just two weeks and it was all shining and new. The staff, half Greek and half British military were superb. We were overjoyed and our little family was complete, at least for the time being. As Jimmy grew and started to toddle he would be welcomed in most of the neighbour's houses. He was very fair haired in contrast to the other children. The locals would take him in and make a fuss of him, his very blond curls were a novelty and often he would come home with tomatoes and grapes, and once he came back with a rabbit in a brown paper bag. I suspect that whoever gave him the rabbit meant for us to make rabbit stew, but John set about making a cage and the rabbit became part of the family. His name was Huey. Occasionally when I took Jimmy to Louis' shop he would be lifted up on to the counter and fed sticky Greek cakes. Eventually he started speaking Greek and when Louis heard it he would roar with laughter. I strongly suspect he was being taught swearwords but I had no way of knowing for sure.

We had been in Limassol for four years when we were posted back to England. We were quartered just outside Weston super Mare in Somerset. I was apprehensive about picking up the reins of my nursing career. Four years seemed a long time to be away. Jimmy had started nursery school so our compromise solution was for me to take a part time staff nurses position. The little seaside cottage hospital was a big change from the large teaching hospital where I had trained. It was small and informal and I thoroughly enjoyed it.

Early in 1969 John came home quite excited with the news that we were to have another overseas posting. By this time Sara had arrived - a tiny, 4lb baby girl. Now our family was complete. It was with a mixture of excitement and apprehension that we prepared for our next posting.

.

Chapter 2

The Berlin years

As a direct contrast to the Cyprus tour, our plane landed at Gatow airport in Berlin in temperatures of minus 20 degrees and thick snow. It was so cold that when I breathed the hairs on the inside of my nose froze and crackled. Thank goodness for efficient German central heating. We were quartered at first in an old Luftwaffe barrack block. It was a series of long corridors divided up into flats and the new arrivals were housed there temporarily for about six weeks. It had a feeling of tube stations during the blitz about it. The old fashioned dark colours of brown, cream and dark green did little to cheer the place up. John started work immediately and I was left with the two children and a feeling of desolation. Those first few days soon passed when I realised that the other wives in the block felt the same and, as in the blitz, it seemed to unite us. Gradually I settled into a regular routine, discovering that there was every facility on the camp and a good and comprehensive social life.

There was a bus stop just outside the entrance to RAF Gatow, and when the weather lifted I would load the push chair on to the bus and go for a jaunt into the centre of Berlin. It was, and still is, a vibrant city. As well as the numerous large department stores stocking everything from pots and pans to gemstones, there was the NAAFI on Theodore Heussplatz, or Naafiplatz, as it was known. Here we could get all the English newspapers although they were a day late and we could also get essentials not found in Germany, like Heinz baked beans and marmite. Not to mention English bread.

I always remember the first time I ventured out of the camp. As I struggled to unload the push chair and keep hold of Jimmy's hand, a lady approached me. She said something in German and I was totally stunned. I know it's ludicrous, but I had expected people to speak English the same as my neighbours in Cyprus. I had a smattering of French from my schooldays but no German at all. I must have conveyed this from my expression because she shrugged, smiled and turned to another passenger. Another time when I took a bus ride to the, 'Big Naafi.' I left Sara's push chair outside. It was easier to carry her than to manhandle it up two flights of stairs. We finished shopping and looked around for the push chair. It was nowhere to be seen. An old German came up and pointed down the road. "Zigeuner," he said. By this time I had enough German to understand that, 'ziguener,' was German for gypsies. Apparently the gypsies had seen my abandoned push chair and made off with it. It was a long hard trek back home on the bus with a load of shopping and two small children in tow.

A little bit about the history of RAF Gatow. It had been a Luftwaffe barracks before the war and was situated on the edge of the West Berlin zone. The nearest neighbours were the East German Peoples National Army - a tank battalion. RAF Gatow was surrounded by wire and the lookout towers could be clearly seen. At the time of the Cold War there was deep suspicion on both sides and the ever present threat from the Soviets. The only way out apart from by air was what known as the corridor. A highly guarded long stretch of road with many checkpoints manned by East German soldiers. The Berlin wall itself was a massive concrete structure with barbed wire and lookout posts dotted around it at frequent intervals and searchlights every hundred yards or so. There was a military train from Berlin to Brunswick. It was heavily guarded, and British troops with guns would patrol up and down the carriages. It was possible to travel through East Germany by car but there were weeks of preparation before making such a journey, it was not to be taken lightly. As well as the checkpoints during which the driver had to get out of the car and queue up with his paperwork. The car was likely to be searched. It was usual for three or four drivers to travel in convoy in case of problems with East German police. Once I even saw a hearse being stopped and searched. That was when I realised that it was no game and that we really were surrounded by hostile forces.

There are numerous stories of people trapped in the east when the wall suddenly went up without warning. Many of them were shot as they tried desperately to escape to the west. Others devised ingenious ways to escape. There were stories of cars being adapted to make room for hidden passengers and babies being hidden under blankets. Soldiers are soldiers everywhere though, and it was common knowledge that Russian cap badges and the fur lined hats were being swapped at the smaller checkpoints, also packs of western cigarettes and other things that were not available in the austere East Germany. Strangely enough, BIC biro pens were much in demand by the soldiers. I think the exchange rate was two Biro pens for one hammer and sickle cap badge.

The currency amongst the British military in Berlin was BAFVs - British Armed Forces Vouchers. They were issued in denominations of 5 to 50 or 100. The American PX (post exchange) dealt in US dollars, the French used francs. Consequently, a trip into town or the US equivalent of the Naafi involved a complicated series of transactions. If we went into Berlin we would have to change our BAFVs into Deutschmarks. If it was a trip to the US base we had to make sure we had dollars, or on the rare outing to the French Economat for perfume or French cheese we needed francs. Just to add to the confusion there were West German and East German Deutschmarks with a vastly differing exchange rate. At the time it was about seven Eastmarks to one Deutschmark.

The camp at Gatow was situated very near the Grunewald, or Greenwood, and the Havel river. It was an idyllic picnic spot and there were cruise boats plying their trade up and down the river. Occasionally we would picnic on the bank or go for a short cruise to Peacock Island. The scenery was out of this world and the peacocks strutted about, their harsh cries could be heard for miles. The Havel is a tributary of the Elbe and provided an important link between East and West Germany. Flowing north it reaches the town of Spandau, infamous for its prison which housed Hitler's deputy, Rudolph Hess, for 36 years. Hess flew solo into Scotland in 1941 in an attempt to negotiate a peace settlement with Great Britain. He parachuted into a field in Ayrshire and was apprehended by a local ploughman who called the Home Guard - shades of 'Dad's Army,' here! He was transferred to the local police station and amid great excitement he was eventually handed over to the intelligence services. He spent the rest of the war years in prison in the UK and was eventually transferred to stand trial at Nuremburg in 1946. Despite pleading amnesia as a defence he was sentenced to life imprisonment which he served at

Spandau. There were several recommendations by the allies for his release after the war but they were continually blocked by the Russian military. Hess committed suicide by hanging himself from a window frame in Spandau prison at the age of 93. There were fears that the building would become a shrine to Neo nazis and it was demolished in 1987 to make way for a supermarket complex which, with typical forces humour became known as 'Hessco's

About every six months or so we would be woken up in the middle of the night by sirens and a loudspeaker mounted on a landrover. This was known as Exercise Rocking Horse. It was a precautionary measure ensuring that all the soldiers and airmen would know the drill if there was ever a Russian invasion. No one knew when this would take place or even if it was an exercise or the real thing. The men would dress hurriedly in their uniforms and rush out to join their units where they would usually hang around for a few hours and then come back home, all fired up and excited. No one got any sleep that night. One memorable night there was a formal dinner at the mess. The revelries went on until 3am. The Station

Commander left at about midnight and we all continued with the dancing and drinking. Staggering into bed at 3.30am, we had just drifted off to sleep when the familiar sound of the siren woke us. Of course, the C.O knew the exercise was scheduled and had the sense to leave the dinner at a reasonable hour.

Every third Sunday there was a large flea market in Berlin. It was near the Brandenburg gate. There were no shops open in Berlin on Sundays but the flea markets were always crowded. The one on 17th June Strasse was vast. Acres and acres of stalls selling everything. There were old Swarovski crystal ornaments, vintage clothing, postage stamps, old post cards, German military medals, though you had to look hard to find a genuine one. The tell tale sign to look for was the medal ribbon. If it showed signs of wear and tear it was more likely to be authentic. There was a large assortment of DDR memorabilia. Russian tools, old vinyl records, Matriyoska dolls, old photographs, lace and linen, slightly motheaten fur coats, and mink hats. Military badges and medals galore. In later years you could even buy a piece of the Berlin wall.

Numerous old oil paintings, perfume bottles, coins - the list goes on.

The German tradition for Kafe und Kuchen - coffee and cake - was one of the pleasant diversions on a Sunday morning. The Konditerai, or cake shops would fill their windows with tempting calorie filled delights. The schwarzwalder kirschtorte, or black forest cherry cake was a favourite. It was so rich I could only manage one piece at a time, though seasoned German housewives could be seen with two large slices and cream on their plate. German ladies can be quite elegant but it has to be said, they are somewhat larger than their French counterparts. French food is for the soul, German food is for the stomach.

As a part of the 'Berlin budget,' a settlement agreed by the allied powers when they partitioned Berlin after the war, service families were allowed certain perks, one of which was a housekeeper. She was paid for out of these funds. Our housekeeper was Mrs Smith or Mrs Schmidt, as she was known. She was a lovely German lady married to a Scotsman. She spoke English with a broad Scottish accent. I had mixed feelings about employing a maid, I felt that there wasn't enough to keep me occupied as I was still unable to work. The housework took up a very small part of my day. Mrs Smith, however, could make housework last for hours. She was thorough and meticulous, as are most German housewives. The children loved her. It was in those years in Berlin with time on my hands that I first started to write.

The large American base at Templehoff used to host frequent barbeques. These were not just small backyard affairs. They were held on a large field with four or five massive braziers. Thick steaks and sausages, copious amounts of beer and lemonade and, of course, burgers and fries, plus an assortment of salads were on offer. There would be entertainers for the children and races with prizes. We all looked forward to these occasions. My German was improving so much that I was confident to go shopping and to try and speak only German. Mostly I managed it. The finer points of grammar would evade me but I could make myself understood.

After two and a half years it was time to move on and we began the laborious process of the 'march out.' Every item of furniture, down to the last teaspoon and light bulb had to be accounted for and the house had to be left spotless for the next occupant. It was a matter of pride that nothing should be less than perfect. We flew from RAF Gatow on a cold November day, arriving at Brize Norton en route to RAF Locking and another adventure.

Chapter 3

UK and the old ladies

By this time I was an old hand at moving and unpacking. As with other military camps, there was everything on the base and I didn't even have to venture into town to fulfil my everyday requirements. There was the ever present Naafi, a library, a post office and most importantly, a primary school for Jimmy, who by this time was 8 years old. Sara was 3 and not yet old enough for nursery. Picking up the threads of my career was out of the question. I could never consider leaving Sara with anyone else. After much discussion and heart searching we arrived at a solution. I would work Friday and Saturday nights with a private nursing agency while John, who was free at weekends, would look after the children. This worked well, and so it was that I enrolled with, 'The West Country Nursing Service.' This was spearheaded by a scatty blonde nurse. Her curly mop of hair was sticking out at angles and her ample chest was straining the buttons on her blouse. She welcomed me with open arms. "Wow! a SRN, we don't get many of those." I was surprised, I had assumed we were 10 a penny.

My first assignment was to care for an old lady of 92. I was supposed to stay overnight, relieving the day nurse. The old lady, Mrs Bolt, had 24 hour care with the agency. There were three of us working shifts. The first one, Glenda, started work at 8am until 5pm, then Alison, a part timer worked from 5 till 9pm. I took over at 9 until 8am. Mrs Bolt lived in a large Victorian town house in Weston Super Mare. It was on a street of similar houses set back from the road. Steps led up to a panelled front door with a gleaming brass knocker in the shape of a lion. Alison opened the door and we introduced ourselves. I had expected a bed ridden patient and was prepared to continue normal nursing care for most of the night. Alison led me through to the sitting room where Mrs Bolt was sitting in a high backed chair by an open fire. "Come here my dear, let's have a look at you." I was a little overawed by her appearance. Regal would fit the description. Her silver hair was piled on top of her head and a jewelled eyeglass on a chain hung round her neck. A massive diamond ring glistened in the light from the fire. "Has

Alison told you my requirements?" She began. Actually Alison had appeared in a hurry to leave and hadn't really said much. "Well," I replied, "Shall we start with you telling me everything you need and I will do my best to supply it." I said brightly. "Oh goody, I see we will get on famously," She said in a plummy voice. "I have my hot milk and whisky at precisely 9.30, then you can help me into my nightgown and tuck me up. Your bedroom is just next door. You will find a bell on the dressing table, should I require anything in the night. My breakfast is served at 7.30 prompt. I have a fresh egg boiled for exactly two minutes and a cup of Earl Grey tea with lemon - never milk," she said. "You will run my bath and when Glenda arrives at 8am she will take over from you." I was dumbfounded. A bedroom! and I was being paid to sleep as well. When I got to know Mrs Bolt a bit more she would tell me snippets of her life in wartime France. She never completed a story and would drift off dreamily halfway through a conversation, leaving me to complete the rest with my imagination. She had been a widow for 30 years and had obviously been left well provided for, as round the clock private nursing was expensive, especially when the old lady wasn't ill. As Glenda said once, a lot of old ladies live in hotel suites, but this way she could stay in her own home and more or less get to choose her nurses. This surprised me because I had assumed nurses were assigned to people without much consideration as to whether they were suitable or not. "Don't you believe it," Glenda said. "If she didn't like you at the first meeting you wouldn't last a day."

My next assignment was totally different, in fact it was a bit unnerving. Mr and Mrs Jarvis were an old couple, both in their 80's. They lived six miles out of town in an old farmhouse. The first night I drove round and round trying to find the place. There were no sign posts and no road signs that I could see. Eventually I found the place. It was difficult to believe that anyone lived there. There was an old rusty tractor in the yard and weeds were knee deep in the muddy drive. I knocked on the door and it was opened by the scruffiest woman I had ever seen. The dirt was caked on her hands and the whole room had a musty smell. She wore a sacking apron smeared with grease. "Who are you?" she asked in a suspicious voice. "I'm the nurse," I replied, trying to smile. She looked vague then suddenly broke into a smile. "Come in, he's in the back," and led me through to what I assumed was the living room. An old man lay on the couch. It was obvious that he was seriously ill. A long bushy beard hid pallid features and his threadbare jacket had holes where the buttons should be. He raised his hand weakly in greeting and fell back on the couch. I had been told very little about this couple. The wife was vague about the details of his illness. "He be old, that's all." She said. I asked what tablets he was taking, hoping that I could find out more of his condition that way. "That doctor come round," she said in her rich West Country accent. "Said he ought to be in hospital but I wasn't having none of that, he's my Joe and I needs him here." I warmed up some soup that was on the iron range and tried to get him to eat some bread with it. Eventually he managed a few crumbs but it seemed to exhaust him. I suggested he would be more comfortable in bed but Mrs Jarvis said he would never manage the stairs, and I was inclined to agree. Settling him down on the couch with blankets and pillows, I prepared to spend the night in an armchair. At about

3am I heard the old woman wandering about. The shuffling noise went on for an hour, then I heard the front door being unbolted. Looking through the farmhouse window I saw Mrs Jarvis in her nightie, ankle deep in mud, crossing the yard. I went to the door and called to her. "I be goin' to feed the chickens," she replied. This was strange as there was no sign of any livestock at all on the farm. "Come back in," I said gently. It had started to rain. "Oh!" she exclaimed, looking bewildered, but she obediently turned around. An hour or so later she was on the prowl again. She appeared at the kitchen door. "Who are you?" she enquired. "I'm the nurse." "What nurse, I don't want no nurse, what are you doing to my Joe?" she said threateningly. It was all I could do to calm her down and persuade her to go back to bed. I was on the edge of my seat for the rest of that night and was glad when morning came and I was relieved by the day nurse. "Oh yes, didn't the agency explain? Mrs Jarvis has dementia, she's quiet most of the time but she can be violent if anyone upsets her." "It would have been useful if someone had told me that," I said ruefully.

My next weekend duty was with another couple of old ladies. It was another large town house, with the same air of faded gentility. Mrs Thomson and Miss Bedford lived together. Apparently Miss Bedford was Mrs Thomson's companion. I wasn't sure what the term, 'companion,' meant, whether it was some kind of paid secretarial thing or whether they were just friends who had drifted together. "We joined forces after the war." Miss Bedford told me. She was obviously devoted to Mrs Thomson. It was a strange setup because Mrs Thomson addressed her more as a servant than a friend. She was an imperious old lady, very genteel in her manner. She was slight and frail and spent most of her time on a red velvet chaise longue. "Hetty dear, would you bring us some tea," she called to Miss Bedford who appeared with a silver tray, delicate bone china cups and a large teapot. "Your duties will be very light," she explained reassuringly. "I need someone to be here in case I become ill." It was obvious to me that she was suffering from heart disease. She had a telltale blue tinge to her lips and was breathless most of the time.

I looked after these two ladies for six months during which time I saw Mrs Thomson deteriorate gradually. She died one morning in December when the snow was deep outside. Miss Bedford was distraught. "I knew she was ill, nurse," she told me, "but I never expected her to go first. I don't know what I'll do now," she sobbed. I heard later that Miss Bedford had died suddenly in her sleep just three weeks after Mrs Thomson. I had grown quite fond of them over the months.

The following week I was assigned to Mrs Maxwell. She was a dear, a widow, her family lived in Australia. Physically she was reasonably well but she had virtually no memory. The GP and Social Services had suggested that she should go into an old people's home but she was very much against the idea. As she said to me once. "I'm not ready for God's waiting room yet." She had been used to cooking for a large family but was now reduced to cooking for one. This was upsetting for her and she showed me her scrapbook of recipes. "Tell you what I'll do, nurse," she said eagerly. "I'll make us a cake." This sounded good so I helped her measure out the ingredients. One by one we weighed out flour, sugar, butter and eggs. The oven was switched on and Mrs Maxwell began to cream the butter and sugar. The energy which was expended put me to shame. She wielded the wooden spoon as if it was a personal vendetta, reducing the eggs to a creamy mass. Eventually the mixture was ready and I turned to the oven. It was cold! Mrs Maxwell had turned it on, I had seen her do it, so what had gone wrong? She had forgotten that she had turned it on and went to turn it on again, obviously turning it off. The cake mixture sat there stagnating as I turned the oven on again. Eventually the cake was cooked though I had to remind her when the cooking time was up. Just before it was time for me to leave I thought maybe I ought to check the kitchen again. Just as well I did because the oven was on full blast and the kitchen was like a hot house.

Another memorable old lady was Miss Frampton, a sprightly 82 year old. The house was large and dilapidated. The remains of what had once been a rose garden surrounded the front entrance. I picked my way through the brambles and rang the door bell. She was an imposing lady, almost six feet tall. Her white hair was tied back with a velvet ribbon. She wore a kaftan in bright colours and copious amounts of eye shadow. Silver photo frames were placed all around the living room. On looking closer I saw that they were mostly of Miss Frampton with recognisable faces from the 1940's and 50's It turned out that she had been an actress and had several roles in the early days of television. She would talk for hours about the old days with snippets of gossip that didn't mean much to me but that she found hilarious.

It seemed at first as if she was name dropping for dramatic effect but when I got to know her I realised that she had actually worked with these famous people. Miss Frampton had an encyclopaedic knowledge of plays and films and could quote line for line from almost anything. She was quite eccentric and I never knew what she was going to do or say next. Her telephone was her lifeline, it rang almost constantly. Long hours were spent reminiscing with the few colleagues and fellow actors that were left. After one of these conversations she would be animated and regale me with tales of theatrical disasters. "Oh, you should have been there, nurse. The curtain wasn't lowered and the corpse was left lying on the stage trying not to move, then, to cap it all, the audience began to laugh." She would shriek with laughter when she told me these stories. I looked forward to my shifts with Miss Frampton.

The night of the hurricane was another memorable one. At 2 o clock in the morning all the lights went out. I have never known darkness like it. Of course, there were no candles or torches anywhere to be found. The wind was howling outside, not just the sounds of a windy night, but a frightening wailing, moaning sound. There were crashes and bangs and the sound of corrugated iron roofs being blown around like twigs. The windows shook and rattled. Miss Frampton appeared in her nightie. "Oh nurse, do something," she wailed. What she expected me to do, I didn't know. "Can you make me a cup of tea?" she asked. With no electricity it was impossible. I had managed to find a lighter and by its faint glow I found a torch. Miss Frampton was terrified. Looking out of the window we could see whole trees bending double in the wind and roof tiles flying by as if they were leaves. "Even King Lear didn't have a tempest like this," she said dramatically. "We shall all die, here and now. It's OK for me, I've lived my life, but you're just a young thing." She had psyched herself up into the role of a dramatic heroine. It was an insight into how she must have appeared on the stage. When the storm died down she remained hyperactive and refused to go back to bed for the rest of the night. As I was leaving the next morning she said brightly "You know, nurse, that was the most exciting thing that's happened for years."

We were waiting for another overseas posting at the end of 1973 so I had gradually tailed off my nursing duties. So it was that when the phone rang one evening I was surprised to be asked to take on just one more job. As the scatty agency nurse put it. "We're desperate, there is no one else." I didn't usually work in the daytime, but what could I do? This time the patient was a man. There had been a family wedding and 'Grandpa' was too ill to attend so someone had to look after him. His daughter answered the door, they were obviously dressed for a wedding. The three grandaughters had identical bridesmaid's dresses and their mother wore the traditional flowy chiffon coat dress and a designer hat. The brother followed behind carrying a box of buttonhole carnations. "Grandpa has his mid day meal at 1 o clock, there is plenty of food in the cupboard, nurse, just help yourself." I was shown into Grandpa's bedroom. He was a charming old man. He was sitting up in a chair wearing a velvet dressing gown. His daughter was anxiously fussing around giving instructions about what he should eat and what time he should have his nap. "Oh, come on, mum," one of the girls shouted. "Grandpa can manage quite well without us nagging him, the taxi is here." They piled out and Grandpa broke into a smile. "That's them out of the way," he grinned. "Go and see what's in the fridge and we'll have ourselves a feast." He sounded like a naughty schoolboy. I got the impression he was enjoying having time away from the family. The fridge was packed full of food, there were family size packs of bacon, dozens of eggs, pots of Cornish cream and large jars of jam. "Well, for a start," he began. "You can forget what Emily said, I don't often get the chance to eat what I want. Can you cook?" I said I could. "So we'll start with bacon and eggs - plenty of bacon, mind," then, "Do you know how to make scones?" I said I could try, and went off in search of flour and butter. Luckily the scones turned out well, which wasn't always the case with my cooking. His sense of fun was infectious and we sat down to a sumptuous meal like two co-conspirators. "There's no need to tell Emily about this," he said. "Now go to the shed out the back and you will find some brandy." I searched the shed and eventually found the brandy hidden behind the flower pots. I didn't join him with his drink although he tried his best to persuade me. I was sent back to the shed to hide the brandy bottle where I had found it. When I came back Grandpa was fast asleep. He slept for the rest of the day snoring loudly. That evening they all returned home from the wedding. Emily, his daughter came in anxiously enquiring if the old man had behaved himself. "Good as gold," I replied and escaped before they could question me further.

Chapter 4

Malta Interlude

Once more it was time to start packing. This time it was Malta. I was quite excited about the posting. The weather in England had been particularly bad so I was looking forward to some sunshine.

We arrived in a thunderstorm. Mediterranean thunderstorms can be spectacular and this one was no exception. Sara was hiding under the back seat of the taxi, 'so that the lightning won't get me.' The street drainage was inadequate to say the least. Rivers of rain water were splashing up over anyone who happened to be standing in the way. The driver didn't moderate his speed for the weather conditions, he drove like a maniac almost cornering on two wheels. Later on I learned that most Maltese drivers drove that way. The rule of thumb for a roundabout was whoever arrives fastest has the right of way. It was rare to go for a week in Malta without witnessing at least three or four accidents.

The forces were returning to Malta after having pulled out, so the married quarters had been left empty. The soft limestone building blocks so prevalent in the Mediterranean attracted damp so, combined with the unpredictable weather it was a breeding ground for mildew. The married quarter was large and my first impression was the musty smell. It smelt cold and damp. Garish carpets and curtains did nothing to add to the ambience and I realised that there was a lot of work to be done to make it into a home. It took about a month of visits to the barrack stores and sweet talking the sergeant in charge. There was no vacuum cleaner, the cooker was temperamental, the taps spurted brown water or none at all. At long last though, I knocked it into some sort of shape. The weather improved and we were reasonably comfortable.

The next thing was to sort out the children's schooling. The forces primary school had just reopened so I took Sara along for a pre school interview. The young teacher sat Sara cross legged on the floor and produced a jar of toffees. Tipping them out, she asked Sara to pick up ten. Sara eagerly counted them out. "That's a clever girl," said the teacher and collected them to put back in the jar. The expression on Sara's face was a mixture of puzzlement and indignation. She thought she would be allowed to keep the sweets. I had to buy some on the way home to pacify her. She took to school like a duck to water. She made friends in her class and in the street where we lived.

As the custom of the time was to work Mediterranean hours - early start and early finish - there was plenty of leisure time for the beach. The sea around Malta is blue and mostly calm. The children learned to swim quickly and would whizz around in their snorkels and flippers. The beach club at Kalafrana was a favourite weekend retreat, we would pack a picnic and spend all day there. There was a shallow swimming pool for the toddlers and a safe swimming area enclosed by a harbour. When the Navy was in port there would be barbecues and parties lasting late into the night. Most ships had a few sailors who could play a musical instrument and there were impromptu concerts. It was an occasion when the big Navy ships sailed into Valetta harbour. The sight was unforgettable. Crowds of people would line up on the ramparts to welcome the ship and cheer the fleet in. The magnificent Ark Royal was an occasional visitor, also the Glamorgan, later to see service in the Falklands.

The social life on Malta was buzzing. When the fleet was in we would go to parties on board ship. The Naval hospitality was legendary and trying to negotiate the crossing from a small pilot boat to a ladder in order to board the ship could be hazardous. Even more hazardous climbing from the boat to the jetty after an evening of rough Maltese wine and Navy rum. It wasn't unusual to have to fish some revellers out of the sea after an evening aboard the Ark Royal. It's sad to think that many of these magnificent ships are no longer in commission.

One of the perks of a posting to Malta was that most families had a cleaning lady. Ours was called Doris. She was short and squat and had a moustache. The children called her Boris behind her back. She was something of a kleptomaniac and often the children's toys would go missing. Once I couldn't find a favourite scarf, only to discover Doris wearing it in town one afternoon. For the sake of peace I simply bought another one the same. I kept a close eye on things after that. Malta is a small island, only about 28 kilometres long by 15 kilometres wide. I asked Doris if she had ever been to the other side of the island. "Oh no. It's too far for me," she replied.

Being surrounded by water the variety of seafood is plentiful. The 'fish man,' would come round in a battered van. Swordfish was a particular favourite. Massive swordfish steaks marinated in white wine with onions was a Sunday treat. The long swords decorated the van, which fascinated the children. They would run behind until it was out of sight. Food shortages on Malta were an everyday occurrence. One week it would be onions, the next week there was no fresh milk so we had to rely on the powdered kind. Potatoes were scarce so we got used to eating rice. It seems strange to reflect that we ate rice then as a necessity in the absence of potatoes, whereas these days rice is an everyday staple. Coffee was difficult to come by and was very expensive so it was a treat when the RAF squadron flew in with large tins of it. Power cuts were frequent so we always kept a supply of candles at hand. It seemed the only thing that was plentiful was bad wine and pizzas. The Italian influence was strong on Malta and there were some good restaurants.

The Maltese are a volatile people and love their fireworks. They have numerous Saint's days and festivals, all accompanied by spectacular explosions. These are not just ordinary fireworks, they are more like small sticks of dynamite. There is very little heed paid to health and safety, indeed it's not unusual to see young men with one or two fingers missing. What with the standard of driving and the casual attitude to safety it's a wonder the population is so dense. On Saturdays and Sundays it seems that the whole population of Malta congregate in the main shopping street in Valetta. It's the highlight of the week to dress in their best finery and walk up and down. Whether they buy anything or not doesn't seem to matter, the object is to be seen.

****

The day the dustbins disappeared. Every Tuesday we would put out our galvanised tin dustbins for collection. As there was no set time for them to be collected we usually put them out the night before. There had been a recent ruling that the people may not put their refuse out in cardboard boxes or plastic sacks because of wild dogs so most of the population had to buy new metal bins. The families living in married quarters had their bins issued from the stores, it was early one morning that the lorry came around to collect the rubbish. The two men in the traditional overalls loaded our bins on to the van and drove off. This was a bit unusual but we thought maybe the bins were being replaced with new modern ones. Two days went by and there was no sign of any new bins. John went to enquire and it turned out that the binmen had no connection to the municipal refuse collectors. That was the last everyone in our street saw of their bins. When we were finally issued with new ones we all stencilled the house number on them in black paint.

The Maltese customs and excise are inclined to be thorough and long delays at the port are commonplace John had decided to drive our car over from the UK. Normally, when alighting from the ship we would have to join a long queue and wait for a minimum of one hour. As it happened, the registration number of our car began with MP. This was a coincidence and bore no relation to the military police. The customs man didn't know this, seeing the registration plate he waved us through and saluted. It took John a little while to work out why.

Malta has a long history going back to the time of the Phoenicians and their architecture reflects this. The walled fortress city of Valetta was home to the Knights of St John, whose cathedral with its magnificent vaulted ceiling and side altars drew visitors from all over the world. Caravaggio's painting. 'The beheading of John the Baptist,' is one of Europe's most impressive works of art. Its dark, brooding atmosphere says much about the artist's troubled state of mind.

The markets in most towns and villages were well worth a visit, especially the fish market in Marsaxlocc. The special Maltese version of fish soup was a favourite. The local fish, lampuki, or dolphin fish was popular too. The market in Mosta town centre attracted hundreds of people, both tourists and residents. The Maltese are creative people, maybe living in a small island has made them self sufficient. We would go up into the hills and see the old women making lace. They would sit in the sun hour after hour making the most delicate and beautiful cloths and pillow cases. I tried it once and failed miserably. Filigree silver is another skill that the Maltese have developed and made their own. Long streets of jeweller's shops in Valetta or Sliema stood side by side with shacks hammering out intricate designs in aluminium or tin. Linen and lace shops competed for space. I bought a green jade Buddha for ten Maltese pounds, only to discover when I got back to UK that it was plastic. It looked authentic though so I still have it.

After just one year in Malta it was time to move on again. This time it was a direct move to Cyprus.

Chapter 5

Cyprus revisited.

Wow Cyprus again. I was over the moon. Not only did we know the island, but as the children were both at school I could think about picking up the reins of my nursing career. As before, the island was in a state of turmoil. This time it was because of the Greek backed military coup. The Greek side of the island was attempting to achieve ENOSIS - union with Greece. That left the Turkish Cypriots out in the cold, so the Turkish army were planning to invade. I began to wonder if it was my destiny to spend my whole life in a war zone. As things turned out, the answer to that was, 'probably.'

As we drove from the airport we passed numerous hastily dug fortifications and random checkpoints. At the time I was unaware of the significance of all this. As before we were housed in a hotel for the weekend. It was a little oasis of calm and the children enjoyed the swimming pool while John went to find out about housing. The situation was much the same, there were many more houses available, most of them with the concrete poles waiting for the second storey. Many of the houses that we had seen in our first visit were now complete, boasting upper floors and even roof terraces.

We settled for a large two storey house near the town in a quarter mainly occupied by British military. Then began the visits to barrack stores for all the essentials to make it into a home. The children raced each other to claim the best bedroom. Sara, being more acquisitive than Jimmy, had her eye on the biggest room but Jimmy, being the oldest declared that it belonged to him. "Mam, tell him, I got here first." "Shut up, squirt. You're only a girl." I had to intervene before it came to blows. "That's for me and your dad so you can look again." I said firmly. The next obstacle was that Sara wanted to paint her bedroom wall in pink and purple. Being a married quarter the things that could be done to personalise our space were limited. We found a compromise by acquiring posters of all her favourite pop stars and sticking them up on the wall with blu tack. We took a trip to Limassol main street which was lined with shops selling everything from leather goods, embroidery, jewellery and sewing materials. I had unpacked my trusty sewing machine and set about making matching curtains and a bedspread in a pattern that Sara chose. Naturally, Jimmy wasn't going to be left out and he chose a scary pattern of daleks and aliens in black and white. The primary school was at Berengaria. It was where most of the children from the street went so the kids settled in well. Now I could think about a job in the medical centre.

****

The Forces Medical Centre in was in Limassol and served the Army, Air Force and attached civilian population. It was manned 24 hours a day and had a team of 6 doctors and 6 nurses as well as RAF medics who covered the evenings and nights. The ambulance drivers were responsible for the upkeep and maintenance of their vehicles so that they were ready at a moments notice for any emergencies. I had been away from main stream nursing for several years so it was a bit hair raising to be thrown back in the deep end. As well as the normal doctor's surgeries there were nurse led clinics for asthma, diabetes and children's ailments. The team of midwives looked after the pregnant mums. The waiting room was always filled to capacity and the team of six nurses would call their patient through one by one. We would deal with the doctor's requests, which could range from syringing a patient's ears to taking blood samples and everything else in between. As well as this we always had a long list of patients who didn't need a doctor, just advice about a child or a dressing. I learned quickly to identify various rashes. I could tell at a glance whether it was measles, rubella or chicken pox. The more obscure viral rashes were slightly more difficult but my confidence grew with time. One milestone was the time I first took blood from a vein. My nurse training had not included this as it was regarded as a task for junior doctors so I was a bit apprehensive. I watched my colleagues taking blood nervously, knowing that sooner or later it would be my turn. I confided in my senior nurse, Jean. She was a plump middle aged sergeants wife. She had been travelling with the army for 15 years and had worked in many service medical centres. She was totally unflappable and I learned a lot from her. "Right," she said. "You can have the next one." She gave me a quick tutorial. "You take blood from a vein, not an artery. If it's dark red you're OK. If it's light and frothy you've hit an artery." This didn't do much for my confidence and I didn't know how authentic her advice was because I had never seen anyone take blood from an artery. Jean told me the exact angle to put the needle in so that it didn't go right through the vein and just how much pressure to apply afterwards to avoid bruising. Nevertheless, seeing is one thing, doing is another. Luckily for me the next patient was a soldier with veins like tram lines. He didn't flinch when the needle went in and the syringe filled up immediately. I was so relieved. I was glad he didn't know that this was my first attempt.

The town of Limassol was in its infancy and there were new buildings going up daily. The local maps couldn't keep up, so it was a nightmare for our ambulance drivers. The local Greek drivers were easiest as they knew the area but the service drivers had great difficulty. It was not unusual to have four new married quarters in a row built on an area which was previously waste ground. The authorities hadn't yet got round to naming the street. Even if the street had a name it would be something unpronounceable in Greek lettering and would not have found its way on to a map.

Emergency calls in Limassol came straight to the medical centre and if they were serious enough they would be transferred to the hospital in Akrotiri. Many of our so called emergencies required nothing more than sticking plaster. We often received 999 calls and here are some examples. "A woman has collapsed in the NAAFI." It was usually a straightforward faint, often from heat exhaustion. "My son has cut his head open." Well, scalps *do* bleed a lot, don't they? On arrival at the scene, blue light flashing we would find a child with a small cut but quite a lot of blood. A steristrip would sort it. "My daughter has swallowed a bead" Time usually resolved this one as nature took its course. There was the occasional high drama when we would have a patient who had been stung by a weaver fish. Though these were not fatal they were extremely painful. There was a tremendous commotion outside the treatment room one afternoon. A young girl of about fourteen was being carried in by her father, we could hear her shrieks up and down the corridor.

"Quick, get a doctor, she's been bitten." Looking at her foot I could see the tell tale three puncture wounds. Quickly picking up a cold spray I gave a quick burst to the affected foot. The effect was immediate. She stopped screaming at once. There was complete silence. Mum and Dad stood open mouthed in amazement. Apparently I had performed a miracle cure. Of course, there were the occasional genuine medical emergency calls. We had just started a shift when the receptionist came rushing through. "Ambulance, quick," she shouted. A lorryload of soldiers had just been overturned on the Akrotiri road. The ambulance driver was waiting with the engine revving when the sergeant medic grabbed me. "Come on Maud, this one is ours." With blue lights flashing and sirens blaring we sped off. Anything in our way would be collateral damage. I clung on to the stretcher in the back, the medic had bagged the front seat. We reached a scene of total devastation There was a two ton lorry on its side, a noisy crowd of locals milling around and ten or so soldiers sitting or lying on the ground. Quickly we assessed the damage. Some were in shock, two had obviously broken bones, and one gave us cause for worry. He was deathly pale and was lying flat out on the ground obviously in great pain. The sergeant medic had years of experience and was able to calm the situation down and reassure the main body of soldiers that now the ambulance had arrived they would all be OK. I admired him for the way he handled this. The men visibly brightened at his approach. We very carefully loaded the injured soldier on to a stretcher after applying a neck brace and decided that, as we were halfway to the hospital anyway there was no point in going back to Limassol. Together we splinted the broken bones, called ahead to the hospital for another ambulance as our land rover could only carry two casualties and sped off in the direction of Akrotiri. Arriving there we were greeted by the waiting trauma team and proceeded to book the injured soldiers in. It was only when I was filling in his details on the admission form that I realised who the injured patient was. He was the husband of a colleague of mine that I knew quite well. I had been so taken up with his injuries and the need to get him to hospital that I hadn't even registered his face. This is just another example of how a nurse can be so involved with an injury that she doesn't recognise the person.

Another interesting 999 call came on new years day 1973. We had been enjoying a quiet day. Everyone else was celebrating and there was a skeleton staff of two nurses, two medics with a doctor on call. The emergency phone blared out and we all jumped. A man had collapsed in Hero's Square and they couldn't wake him. Hero's Square is the rather sordid quarter of Limassol where all the dubious brothels were reported to be. Every military garrison town has one of these areas. It was known as, 'the gut' in Malta, Hero's Square in Cyprus and Bugis Street in Singapore. Not knowing what to expect I grabbed the medic and we roared off, screeching to a halt outside a dimly lit bar. Two or three soldiers accompanied us inside and there, on the floor was a deeply unconscious Scotsman in full regalia. Kilt, sporran and all. As I leant over to check his pulse I caught a whiff of pure Scottish whisky. The man was paralytic. As the medic and the other soldiers lifted him on to the stretcher I caught a full on glimpse of what a Scotsman wore (or did not wear) under his kilt. Apparently he had been celebrating Hogmanay since midnight and it was now 2pm. We loaded him on to the ambulance and made our way back to the medical centre, this time at a more sedate pace. The soldier, who had been deeply unconscious, woke up just as we were reaching the medical centre. He flatly refused to come inside and see the doctor. He became aggressive, aiming a punch at the medic No amount of persuasion on my part could get through to him. I went inside to tell everyone what was going on and our warrant officer, an old sweat with some twenty years service said, "leave this to me sister." He came back to the ambulance with me, saluted the Scotsman on the stretcher and said, "the medical officer requests that you come inside immediately." The transformation was amazing. He sat bolt upright, saluted back and allowed us to escort him inside. Afterwards I asked the warrant officer how he had managed it. "It was the word 'officer,' that did it." He grinned. "These Scottish regiments are all disciplined and experienced soldiers, it's ingrained in them. If I had just said, 'the doctor wants to see you,' it would have had no effect." I learned something new that day as well as what a Scotsman wore under his kilt.

We had all had our photographs taken for a notice board to go in the waiting room along with a mission statement, which was the latest buzz word going around. Things were changing and everything was becoming more corporate with care plans and foot long faxes detailing all the changes taking place. We had a good team of nurses in Limassol. We all got on well and would congregate in the dispensary when it was quiet. Sandy, one of the younger nurses had a tremendous sense of humour, she could make a joke about anything. One morning I walked into dispensary and found them all rolling about laughing. Sandy had found a huge poster of girls in various stages of undress and had superimposed photos of each of us on the heads of these bodies. There was me in black stockings and suspenders and little else. Sandy had on a red basque, the other girls had various thongs and tassels. This poster remained behind the door for a few weeks. As no one else came into the dispensary except the nurses, we weren't too concerned, but inevitably the news got around and there were visits from a few curious doctors and medics who came to have a look

All the time there were rumblings about a Turkish invasion. With a, 'head in the clouds', attitude we assumed it wouldn't happen. Only when the neighbours over the road started building trenches in their back garden did we begin to wonder. Even then we thought that somehow it would pass us by. John came home one Friday with news that all the families in Limassol had been advised to keep in supplies of food to last twentyfour hours. The NAAFI, never very well stocked, soon ran short of tinned supplies. The local Greek supermarkets that had recently sprung up stocked more tins of food but as we could not read the Greek alphabet we had to rely on the pictures on the tins. The families living on the camp at Akrotiri were briefed as to what would happen in the event of an invasion. They were advised to keep any spare rooms free to accept families from the Limassol quarters on a temporary basis until they could all be evacuated back to UK.

One incident that sticks in my mind from that time concerns a local Greek army check point just outside Akrotiri. We were driving along with the children in the car when Sara dropped her toy dog out of the window. She set up such a yell that John stopped the car and went back to retrieve it. When we reached the check point the Greek soldier, instead of waving us through as he would usually do, stopped us and motioned us to wind the window down. He poked his gun through and barked "Why did you stop the car?" John reached out, calmly pushed the rifle aside and showed him the toy dog. I was terrified! The soldier didn't quite know what to do. He didn't want to lose face and he had expected John to be intimidated by the gun. Glancing around at his colleagues, he said menacingly "Well, don't stop the car again...Sir."

Work went on as usual in the medical centre and the social life didn't suffer. Most afternoons we would pile into our little Fiat 500 and drive down the bumpy track to Governor's beach on the Dekhalia road. The blue waters went on for miles and the sand was clean and golden. It was shallow for about half a mile out and the children learned to swim and snorkel. Sara, at the time was tiny and her flippers were almost as big as she was. She would flip along like a fish and we had to watch her carefully as the flippers would propel her along faster than we could swim to catch her. Another favourite excursion was a trip to the Troodos mountains. The great snow capped Mount Olympus was a magnificent sight and we could feel the air growing cooler and fresher as we drove up higher. Cyprus, though small, is an island of contrasts, from the blue Mediterranean beaches to the craggy uplands the scenery is always breathtaking.

As well as Governors beach, another favourite haunt was Happy Valley on the Episkopi camp. It was reached via a steep incline and the shoreline was more rocky than Governors. There were more long stretches of golden sand and the bonus of several shacks selling cold drinks and ice cream. Aphrodite's rock loomed majestically out of the sea, the legendary site where in Greek mythology, Aphrodite, the goddess of love and the mother of Eros, was born out of the sea foam and floated ashore on a sea shell, as depicted in Botticelli's, 'The Birth of Venus.' Legend has it that under certain weather conditions the waves form a column of water that dissolves into a pillar of foam resembling an ephemeral human form. Anyone fortunate enough to witness this will meet the right person very soon. The salt flats on the way to Akrotiri base were home to hundreds of flamingos. To see them all with their pink plumage was a sight to remember. Hundreds of yards of pure colour. It was breathtaking.

There were clapped out and decrepit buses serving most of Limassol. They ground along and you could hear them coming for miles. Brightly coloured with various religious artefacts dangling from the windscreen, they would screech along. They were always crowded. There would be local farmers complete with a goat or two and several chickens. Black clad housewives with wicker baskets full of produce from the market. The old men would strap their bicycles on the back of the bus and jump on board. More than once I saw the bus drive off leaving an irate farmer without his bike stranded by the road. As I didn't drive at the time I used to catch the local bus if I wanted a trip to Limassol town. The driver always wore a flower behind his ear. He got to know where all his regular passengers lived and would often toot his horn outside our house to see if I was going into town. The kids would shout, "mam, here's flower ear's bus." I suppose there were organised bus stops somewhere but nobody took any notice of them. If you wanted a bus you just stood in the road and held up your hand. The bus would pull up sharply and it was just bad luck if anyone happened to be driving too close behind.

Another memory was our wedding anniversary. We called a taxi to go to a well known fish restaurant on the sea front. There were the usual crowds of people milling around and an old man on a bicycle was weaving in and out of the traffic. Suddenly he turned right without signalling and our taxi clipped the edge of his bike. The poor old man was thrown on to the road and within minutes he was surrounded by gesticulating Greek men. I tried to get them to leave him flat until the ambulance came, but as I was only a woman nobody took any notice. He was hauled to his feet, pale and shocked and in obvious pain. He was loaded on to a passing lorry and headed to the Greek hospital. Within a couple of days two Greek policemen came to our house to get a statement about the incident. They asked John how fast he estimated the taxi to be going and his view of what had happened. It turned out that the taxi had practically no brakes. I hope the old man had adequate compensation

Sofoulla, our original landlady, was married by this time and she came to visit occasionally with her new baby, Andreas. He was gorgeous with a mop of curly jet black hair and eyes as black as liquorice allsorts. She was so proud of him and regaled me with details of her labour from the first twinge to the delivery in graphic detail. At that stage John made a tactical withdrawal

The day we went to a Greek wedding sticks in my memory A young friend of ours had married a local Greek girl and we were all invited. To say it was different was an understatement. First of all, instead of sitting politely in the church as we would normally do, everyone was milling around laughing and talking while the priest in his high black hat and robes intoned the ceremony. Martin and Maroulla had garlands on their heads and she looked beautiful in an elaborate costume and professional make up. Sparkling brown eyes heavily lined with kohl. When the actual wedding ceremony was over we all adjourned to a highly ornate room at the back of the church. There were at least a hundred and fifty guests crammed into a fairly small space. As the new couple moved among the crowd the custom was for them to make three circuits of the room and then all the guests would pin money on to their clothes, then the dancing and fun would start and last well into the night. The cutting of the cake was a bit of a surprise Martin, the groom and Maroulla held the knife and proceeded to cut the first layer. The knife went through smoothly enough until it reached the base of the cake. They sawed, pushed and hacked, to no avail. It appeared that the bottom layer, instead of icing, was plywood covered with white icing. Lifting the two top layers off they discovered that all of the separate layers had a base of plywood

Greeks are hospitable people and it's customary if anyone crosses your threshold to offer them either food or drink. YaYa was an old lady of about eighty or more. I was attempting to tidy the garden when she appeared at my gate. 'May I have a drink?' she said in Greek. My Greek wasn't too good but I gathered from her gasping motions that she was thirsty and about to expire. I invited her in and filled a tumbler of iced water from the fridge. She looked at it, paused, and said, "coca cola." If I had thought eighty year old grannies liked coke I would have offered it first. She was a frequent visitor after that, so I kept a supply in the fridge.

Our Greek landlord took to visiting to inspect the house, usually when John was in work. He would accompany me from room to room and when we reached the bedroom he would look at me lasciviously and say, "when more babies?" I would smile and say, "two is enough," but something in his manner made me feel uncomfortable. We decided to move to another house nearer my work at the medical centre. As landlords were always looking for tenants, the 'to let,' signs went up immediately. One Sunday afternoon John and I were snoozing in the bedroom. As it was high summer we weren't wearing much. Suddenly a Greek family appeared in the room. Mama, Papa and three black eyed children. To say we were surprised wouldn't cover it. They had been passing and seen the Enoikiazetai - 'To let' - sign. Assuming the house was unoccupied, they had come to have a look. Cyprus in the '70's was quite informal and this wasn't unusual behaviour.

About this time we acquired a kitten. Scruffy was his name. He was a tiny tabby and would follow Sara around. That is, until the day he disappeared. We searched everywhere, put up notices, but there was no sign of him. Sara was distraught, but with the resilience of children, she soon forgot about him. About a month later she came rushing in. "Mam, mam, I've found Scruffy but he won't come out." We all went to look and found him, stiff as a board and quite dead inside a water pipe in the back garden. He had obviously crawled up there and been unable to get out. Jimmy made up some story about the water pipe being the way to cat heaven and thats where Scruffy is now. It seemed to pacify Sara.

Mrs Nicolaides who lived across the road had four daughters and we would regularly see four or five lines of washing blowing in the breeze. A knock came at our door and it was one of the daughters, Electra. She had heard that we were planning to move and wanted to know if we were going to sell our washing machine. I thought about it and decided that we would buy a new one for when the tour of duty ended, and take it home with us. I quoted a price which I thought was reasonable for the machine as it was working perfectly. Again, I hadn't factored in the Greek custom of bargaining. So it was that that I sold it for half the price I had planned. John went over to their house to install it and the family all crowded around to see it in action. John explained all the technical details to Ioannis, the husband - the women wouldn't understand! A few days later I was in the garden and saw Mrs Nicolaides lugging a basket of wet washing from the backyard into the kitchen. I later discovered that before loading the washing machine she would first wash everything by hand. So much for labour saving devices.

Our time with the forces was rapidly drawing to a close. After ten years spent mostly overseas we had had many adventures and an exciting life, but had no fixed base in England. The big decision had to be made. Do we continue our travelling abroad or do we settle down and find a permanent job where we could buy a house and provide some stability. The children were approaching the stage when they needed some continuity in their education. It was a time for much discussion. We had travelled all our married life and the thought of settling down was worrying. As well as these stresses, the Greek/Turkish situation was gathering pace. We were now on amber alert on a fairly permanent basis. The NAAFI continued to struggle to provide for a siege situation. The medical centre had a huge increase in stress related illnesses and even the children came home from school asking when the aeroplanes were going to bomb us. As it turned out, our tour in Cyprus ended early in 1974 and we missed the Turkish invasion by three months.

Early in 1974 a Greek led military coup deposed the president, Archbishop Makarios and installed Nicos Sampson, a military man, in favour of ENOSIS, union with Greece, in his place. Rumours abounded that Makarios had been killed, but actually, he escaped first to the Sovereign base area at Akrotiri and thence to Malta, en route to London. In response to this, the Turks invaded Cyprus on 20th July 1974. It was a brief and bloody conflict. They landed at Kyrenia and fought their way towards Famagusta. The military families based at Famagusta were evacuated in a convoy of trucks to the Limassol end of the island before being flown back to UK escorted by Lightning jet planes in case of Turkish threat to their air space.

The Sovereign base area at Akrotiri was opened to families of refugees fleeing from the Famagusta and

Kyrenia end. As with any exciting event, some urban legends grew up, not least of which was the ?apochryphal? story of the Commanding officer of the Royal Regiment of Fusiliers who drove his land rover to a crossing point and stood in the middle of the road to deter the Turkish tanks. Also there was the story of the Turkish tank which drove on to the SBA at Ayios Nicolaos when it ran out of fuel. According to legend the British refuelled it and sent it on its way. By the time these events occurred we were in rented accommodation in UK while looking around for somewhere permanent to call home.

Chapter 6

Resettlement blues

Late '74 to '75 was a stressful time for the whole family. We had left the secure environment of the forces where every whim was catered for. If I needed a new cooker I would simply phone the barrack stores and it would be provided. The same applied to furniture and fittings, down to the last curtain hook or light bulb. The NAAFI was just around the corner and the school was within walking distance. The ongoing political tension seemed to pass us by and there were very few worries. We realised, however that the time had come to move on.

We flew from Akrotiri to Brize Norton as a family. As the plane gathered height over Cyprus we could see the snow capped peaks of mount Olympus through the porthole window. Sara said, "bye bye, Cyprus," and for some reason my eyes filled with tears.

Landing at Brize Norton late in the afternoon we decided to stay the night nearby and arrive rested and refreshed at my sister's house in Wales. Our car was waiting for us when we got off the plane as John had had it shipped back to UK previously. It was a relief to see it standing there. I looked at John and the children and it suddenly dawned on me. Here we were in England. No home, no job and no ever ready support from the military community. It was a daunting moment. John had terminal leave from the Air Force so his salary was coming in for the next two months, which gave us some breathing space.

Arriving at my sister's house in Wales all the relatives crowded in to see us, we were something of a novelty. It was lovely to see everyone and remark on how they had all grown and hear all their news over two or three bottles of duty free wine. After a week we went to stay with John's mother while we did a trawl round the local estate agents. We quickly discovered that cramming a family of four into a very small house was a potential minefield and we took a short let on a holiday house in Cheddar, Somerset. Before we left the forces John had been writing to various firms enquiring about jobs but the response was slow. I settled the children temporarily in the local school in

Cheddar and took a part time job in a tourist cafe′. This meant that I had access to the magnificent Cheddar caves. Sara thought it was like fairyland with all the hidden lighting showing up the stalactites and stalagmites.

In the meantime John was in Wales looking at houses. We settled on a four bedroomed house on a new estate. We all trooped down to view it and decided that it had everything we needed at the moment. Next was a visit to the bank to arrange a mortgage. The sharp suited mortgage broker ushered us in to a plush office where we were offered coffee and biscuits. The interview began. We felt it was going fairly well until the young man asked John where he worked and if he could provide evidence of regular employment. There was a silence, then John replied, "I don't actually have a job at the moment, I am on terminal leave from the forces." The young man's face altered just fractionally, the corporate smile slipped a millimetre as he saw his commission disappearing. "I'm afraid we must have evidence of current employment before I can proceed any further," he said. "We will, of course, keep your application on file." And that was that.

That same afternoon John went to a local factory that manufactured and assembled hearing aids. Being an experienced engineer he was offered a job immediately and came home triumphant. The pay wasn't brilliant but at least it was a job. The next visit to the bank was more fruitful and with our gratuity payment from the forces as a deposit we obtained a mortgage. Thing were looking up. There followed a frustrating and anxious four weeks while we waited for the contract to be drawn up and signed and completion to take place. After what seemed like an interminable time we were at last handed the keys to Rolls Avenue. We said our goodbyes to Cheddar and piled in the car. At last we had a roof over our heads and some degree of security. It had been a long and difficult three months. We were now the owners of a four bedroomed detached house costing £9000. That first evening we sat around an old camping table on plastic chairs and ate a take away meal. The children slept on green canvas fold up army beds and John and I shared a mattress on the floor. Tomorrow would begin the hunt for furniture.

We had been window shopping for months but now we were free to actually choose some furniture. I had had my eye on sofa and chairs and had been staking out the shop for weeks, hoping it hadn't been sold. Early on the morning after we had moved in I went scurrying down to the furniture shop, breathing a sigh of relief that my chosen sofa was still in the window. What a disappointment! It appeared that there was an eight week waiting list for that particular model. In spite of my impassioned pleas and my painting a pitiful picture of a family living off plastic chairs, the salesman wouldn't budge. "But you have it there in the window." I moaned. "Yes madam, but if we were to sell that model there would be nothing to advertise, so we couldn't sell any more of them." This turned out to be the pattern for most of the furniture I wanted to buy, including beds and dining tables. Even carpets proved difficult. On reaching home I sat down and cried. I just wasn't used to having to wait. What a lot I had to learn!

John came up with the solution. "What we'll do," he said is search through the small ads in the local papers, people are always buying and selling furniture.

We can furnish the house in a couple of days, while we wait for your sofa and chairs. When everything is ready we can resell the old stuff." Trust John to come up with a workable solution. He was always more practical than me. Fortunately we managed to get carpet for the whole house within a couple of days so it was all ready to receive the furniture, We acquired an old but very comfortable three piece suite, a couple of bunk beds and a large dining table. Now it was beginning to look like home. Then came the hunt for curtains, blinds, lampshades, crockery, cutlery, table linen and hundreds of other items that we had never had to buy before. They got to know me at the local department store.

The garden presented a problem. Because it was a new estate, the back garden was just bare earth with a few bricks and boulders buried underneath the topsoil. I knew nothing about gardening and it was a steep learning curve. It seemed that the only things that grew in abundance were weeds. My neighbour advised against putting weed killer down if I ever wanted to grow flowers or vegetables. Consequently a large part of my time was spent digging and pulling up dandelions.

The children were used to frequent moves and settled in to the new school well. Jimmy was something of a novelty in his class because of his English accent. Inevitably, the other kids wanted to know all about him, where he came from and where he stood in the pecking order. When he explained that he had moved around and been to several different schools and couldn't really say where he came from he earned the nickname, 'everywhere.' This was reinforced, rightly or wrongly, by his teacher. I think, secretly, Jimmy was proud of it. It rained for all of the first five weeks and the roads around the estate were knee deep in mud. Sara, aged six, was picking her way home from school through the building site when she got stuck in the mud. Tom, one of the builders we had got to know picked her up, put her on his shoulders and delivered her to our door. It was a more innocent age then, nowadays it's unlikely that would happen.

During that time the Welsh Valleys were in the grip of a recession. Firms and factories were closing down with frightening regularity. John could see the writing on the wall and began looking for a more secure job. Computers were in their infancy and the latest new gadget was called a facsimile machine, known universally now as a fax machine. John went on a course to learn how these worked and due to his experience with communications in the forces, he was offered the job of communications engineer for West Wales. This was a huge step up from hearing aids, but it involved a lot of travelling. As at that time there were very few offices in Wales that actually possessed a fax machine, his area stretched eventually over much of the UK. He would stay in hotels while travelling the West Country, repairing and installing the machines. Occasionally, in the school holidays, he would take Jimmy along with him. I was left at home with Sara, still struggling to maintain the garden. This was not how it was supposed to be! When we were in the forces I expected him to be away occasionally, but this was different. There I had a support network. Gradually I made friends and Angie, a lady who lived across the road with children the same age as mine, became a good friend and a mine of information. I began to settle in.

When the children were settled in school I began to wonder about the possibility of getting a part time job. Nursing was out of the question because the hospital was some miles away and I would have had to work shifts. This wouldn't have fitted in with school hours. There was a new Carrefour supermarket opening up locally and they were advertising for staff. I decided to go for an interview. Dusting off my only smart suit I went off to be interviewed. I was ushered in to a small ante room with three other girls and eventually the receptionist called me through for the interview. It was much larger and there was a large desk dominating the room Four men sat the other side of it and there was a chair in front for me. I studied the four men in their business suits. One sat at the side with a clip board and another one - his suit was a better cut - sat at the desk. The other two appeared to me to be a bit nondescript and so I didn't remember many details about them, except that they all seemed to defer to the man in the middle.

I thought privately that this was rather high powered for just a shop job. Obviously they didn't agree. There was a barrage of questions, for example.

"What do you think you can bring to the job?" I replied, "Experience with people, a professional qualification and common sense." This was duly noted by the man with the clipboard. The next question was, "would you be prepared to travel?" This surprised me, the shop was less than a mile away. Of course I wouldn't be prepared to travel. The turning point for me came for me when I was asked, "is your family complete?" Of course I considered my family to be complete but it was none of their business, and I implied that without exactly putting it into words. After several more questions, many of which I considered irrelevant they asked me if there was anything I wanted to ask. As they hadn't mentioned salary I said, "I would like to know, if I am offered the job, and if I take it, what will the salary be?" They seemed a bit taken aback. Apparently most interviewees left that question out. This surprised me, as surely the reason for taking a job as opposed to a profession or a calling, is money. "You will be starting at a salary of 50 pence per hour," the man in the good suit said. My jaw dropped. Before I could stop myself I said, "that's not a lot." Hurriedly he continued. "There will be opportunities for promotion if you apply yourself." How supercilious he sounded. I left the interview full of indignation and headed straight to Angie's house for coffee and a post mortem. Strangely, she didn't consider 50 pence per hour to be a bad wage. What planet was she on? I determined that when the letter came offering me the job I would take great pleasure in refusing it. In the event, I need not have bothered. Two days later I received a letter in the post.

Dear Mrs Harris

We regret we are unable to offer you a position at this time. We will, however, keep your details on file.

I didn't know whether to be relieved or indignant.

I was just beginning to feel at home in the new surroundings, the children had made friends and the garden was seventyfive percent sorted. There was still the nagging inconvenience of having to deal with all the mundane everyday things without John there most weekdays, when the bombshell fell. He breezed in one Friday and I could feel the barely suppressed excitement radiating from him. "How do you feel about another overseas posting?" "You're joking," was all I could manage to say.

It appeared that one of the many job applications that he sent out while we were in transit between the forces and, 'civvy' street, had borne fruit. And what delicious fruit it was! British Forces Broadcasting Service, or BFBS, had come up with an interview for a broadcasting engineer. The location wasn't mentioned but we knew that as well as the headquarters in London and Chalfont st Giles, there were dozens of overseas opportunities available. BFBS broadcasts to the forces wherever they may find themselves. It is a link with home, known and appreciated by most serving soldiers. I didn't need to be asked twice. I was euphoric. Settling down in one place was one thing, but being able to travel and enjoy the lifestyle we had known was too good an opportunity to miss. We now owned a house, so even if things went wrong we would have somewhere to come back to. Also, we could let the house and it would pay the mortgage. It seemed like a win win situation. John breathed a visible sigh of relief. "I thought you might not want to uproot us all again," he said.

When the children came in from school we sat them down and sounded them out about a possible move. To my great relief they were as enthusiastic as I had been. Then came the day of the interview. John went on the train up to London and there followed an anxious couple of days while we waited. On the third day the phone rang and John was told he had passed the interview board and was provisionally offered a post with BFBS as a broadcasting engineer. A letter with all the details would follow. He drove straight to the off licence for a bottle of champagne.

The letter duly arrived in the post After a period of orientation in London, starting in one month's time there was a strong possibility of a posting abroad. The next day I went rushing over the road to tell Angie our news. She couldn't take it in. "But you've only been here five minutes," she said, "And what about the house?" All these things I had discussed with John the previous evening. To anyone who has never travelled it must have seemed daunting, but we were well used to that lifestyle. The next step was to tell the family. "Well," my aunt said. "I said we'd give you six months before you up sticks again, and I was right, wasn't I?"

The next month was spent preparing for a move. As we hadn't been given a posting yet there was not too much we could do to prepare. John gave notice to the fax machine firm and took up the orientation post in London, coming home on weekends. At the end of the first week he came home with tremendous news. The job was one he had dreamed of and there was talk of an engineer post in Singapore. "Don't build your hopes up," he told me. "It sounds almost too good to be true." At the end of the orientation period the director of engineering called him in to the office. "Well, John, you seem to have fitted in seamlessly. We are impressed with your level of expertise in what is essentially a new field." John didn't consider it a new field, communications was his background as well as his passion. "What would your wife think about a posting to Singapore?" "You wouldn't have to ask her twice," he replied.

The next three months flew by. There was packing and storage to arrange, deciding whether or not to sell the car - as it happened, arrangements were in place to ship it to Singapore - which helped a great deal. We visited the estate agent to arrange to let the house and made visits to both sets of relatives before we embarked on this latest adventure. We were quite worried initially as there were no replies to our advertisements to let the house and time was getting short. Then, miraculously when there was just three weeks left, an estate agent rang. By coincidence, a Chinese man and his family had just arrived in England and were looking for a place to live. Mr Chang worked in a restaurant in town and he had just brought his wife and three sons over from Thailand. So it was that, as we flew to Singapore, Mr Chang's family flew to Wales. Things were looking up.

The day before we left I went around to the office of the building site to say our goodbyes and to thank the men for their friendliness and help. The foreman offered me tea in an enamel mug. He expressed surprise that we were packing up and moving after less than a year. "Well, Bill, it's only bricks and mortar." I said. I felt there were better things on the horizon, and I was right.

Chapter 7
Exotic Singapore.

Once again we flew from a cold UK to another hot climate. We stopped to refuel at Gan in the Indian Ocean. The stopover was about an hour and we revelled in the lush greenery all around us. There were huge fruit bats hanging upside down from the trees, they were about the size of kittens. Palm trees surrounded us, it was like paradise. All too soon we had to board the plane for the onward leg of our journey.

Landing at Changi airport in Singapore the hot and humid air enveloped us. It literally wrapped itself around us as we boarded the mini bus to take us to the Premier Hotel. We were to spend two weeks there while our married quarter was made ready. Needless to say, with a huge swimming pool, the children were over the moon. We had barely entered our air conditioned room when Sara upended a suitcase searching for her bathing costume. Jet lag didn't seem to affect the children, though John and I felt in need of an afternoon sleep.

While John went to the BFBS studios I had the life of a lady of leisure. Sara and I explored the long street of shops. There was colour everywhere, from the sari's worn by the local ladies to the brilliantly painted temples and exotic birds and flowers Singapore was a riot of colour and exotic smells. The jewellery shops took my breath away. There were rows and rows of massive rubies, emeralds and diamonds. All at prices we considered unbelievably cheap. At any hour of the day or night there was something going on in Singapore. In the evenings the car park on Orchard Road would be cleared and the *makan* stalls would be set up with hawkers selling all manner of exotic foods. There was chile crab, chicken, complete with head and beak, portions of snake cut like steaks, Peking duck, which we could smell twenty yards away. Fruit was piled high, long sticks of bananas fresh from the palm tree, lychees, passion fruit, pineapples, prickly pears and the dreaded durian, which tasted like heaven and smelled like hell. One of the more famous of these eating stalls was, 'Fatty's,' in Albert street. The proprietor was immense, he obviously enjoyed the food he cooked. We could get any dish we wanted at Fatty's, but his speciality was chile crab. The stall was in the open air and the locals would throw their discarded chicken bones and crab shells on the ground where they would be whisked away by the rats. Strangely enough, the only bout of 'Ghandi's revenge' we ever suffered was due to prawns bought in a smart and prestigious shop on Orchard Road. On a nostalgic visit back to Singapore some thirty years later, Fatty's was still there although it was now run by his son. It had become sanitised and the prices had quadrupled.

Back in the '70s many poorer Malay families lived in kampongs, settlements crowded together like so many shanty towns. Whole families crowded into two small rooms. The cooking facilities were primitive so most local Chinese ate at these food malls. Lee Kwan Yew, the prime minister was aiming to bring modernisation to the city. One by one the kampongs were being replaced by blocks of flats. There were daily reports of 'accidental' fires in the kampong areas. The inhabitants would then have to be rehoused.

Singapore was the cleanest city I had ever encountered due to the draconian laws imposed on all the population. There were fines for every breach of hygiene, for example, there was a fine for spitting in the street. It didn't seem to apply to the older Chinese men around the downtown market. There, we would have to jump aside to dodge them. It wasn't wise to come between an old Chinese grandpa and his spitoon! Laws against dropping chewing gum or litter were rigidly enforced. They even had, and still have, corporal punishment in the form of the rotan - a bamboo cane. As the population of Asia continued to grow the government introduced a law stating that Singaporean couples should only have one child. Notices were displayed in the post office and most government buildings proclaiming in large black letters. "Boy or girl, one is enough." Also the seventies saw the tail end of the hippy movement in America and Europe. This was felt as a threat by the powers that be, and more notices were placed in government buildings. "Persons with long hair will be served last."

Every week there was a large thieves market on Sungei road. This had been in place for years and flourished in the late '60s after the British withdrawal. Military equipment and uniforms, usually looted, were readily available. If a house had been burgled, a not infrequent occurrence, one could often go to the thieves market and buy back ones own possessions. The vendor would deny all knowledge of where he obtained the goods. It was common to make a purchase on the Friday, and by the Saturday the vendor would have disappeared. Also along the Sungei road were the opium dens, crumbling houses where elderly opium addicts eked out their time. They were known as, 'death houses.' Further along were hundreds of stalls selling Chinese medicine. Their pungent smells were easily recognisable. The sellers purported to have remedies for every ailment whether physical or psychological. There was rhino horn as an aphrodisiac, sets of acupuncture needles, illustrated charts showing how the human body worked and herbs for every ailment known to man. We supposed some of them may be effective as the stalls were always crowded with customers.

The climate was hot and humid all the year round, with the monsoon season round about Christmas time.

There would be two or three days of unbearable humidity, then the sky would turn purple and the rain would come. Not just ordinary rain, but great deluges often accompanied by spectacular thunder and lightning. Monsoon drains about three feet deep were dug alongside every road and when it rained they would fill up in half an hour. It was not unusual for unfortunate locals to slip and drown in one of these drains, the current of rushing water being too strong for them to escape.

After two weeks in the hotel our married quarter was ready. What a revelation! It was by far the biggest house we had ever lived in. Set in a tree lined estate of similar houses occupied by the Diplomatic Service and the military, it was palatial. Cane furniture, marble floors and a sweeping staircase up to the bedrooms. My first impressions left me speechless. Was all this luxury ours? Not only that, we had a live in Amah, a kind of maid- of- all -work, and a gardener. We also inherited a dog. It was customary among the expatriates in Singapore, when they returned to UK to leave the staff for the next occupant. Talk about a colonial lifestyle - we were living it! Siti, our amah lived in a small room attached to the house, she had her own furniture and was quite self sufficient. She was about fifty years old and had been an amah for years serving many British families. There wasn't much she didn't know and I learned a lot from her. She spoke a mixture of Malay and broken English. I decided after a while that I would like to learn to speak Malay. I went into town, bought a book on grammar and went rushing back to Siti to ask her if she would help me. She looked crestfallen and replied, "mem, Siti no go to school, Siti no learn to read." She always addressed me as 'mem,' short for memsahib, and John as tuan which, in Malay, means master or boss.

We had frequent dinner parties, as BFBS were a sociable crowd. This is where Siti came into her own. If we didn't have enough cutlery or crockery for a large group she would liase with the other amahs, they had their own network, and miraculously, silver cutlery would appear. It would be returned the next day to whatever family they had borrowed it from.

Large French windows looked out on to a huge garden with orchids, palm trees and - our pride and joy - one lone pineapple. We watched it grow for a whole season, the children giving us daily reports on how big it had become. "When will it be ready to eat?" Sara asked almost every day. She grabbed Siti by the hand and led her to the garden to report on its progress. "Pineapple ready in four days," said Siti, holding up four fingers. Early on the morning of the fourth day Sara and Jimmy got up at 7am, and went rushing into the garden in their pyjamas. "Can we pick it, mam?" John came out with a knife and proceeded to cut the pineapple down. We took it inside ceremoniously. Disaster! When we opened it up we saw that the whole interior had been eaten away by red ants.

As well as red ants, Singapore hosted dozens of other creepy crawlies. There were snakes, scorpions, stag beetles, butterflies as big as dragons, to name just a few. There was a brain fever bird. I think it was a mynah bird. He could imitate the ring of the telephone to perfection. Many times we would rush to answer it and discover that it was the pesky mynah bird. The golden oriole was another inhabitant of our garden, along with a family of jays and numerous others that I couldn't identify.

The children had settled in to school, Jimmy at the secondary school and Sara at still at the primary. Every Thursday was food shopping day and I would bring in the supplies for the week. Jimmy had made a friend in school and most Thursdays he would wander over from the other side of the camp. I didn't think much about this, I just accepted that he was Jimmy's friend, but Siti was wise to the ways of the world. She wouldn't say outright that she disliked this lad, but by the odd sniff and toss of her head when he came knocking on the door we gathered that she wasn't impressed. Eventually I asked her why she didn't like him. "He only come on shopping day," she replied. "No biscuits and sweets, he no come." I decided it was worth a few biscuits and sweets for Jimmy to have a friend. Michael and Jimmy got into a lot of mischief together, teasing Sara and generally annoying Siti. One afternoon I came in and there was a strong smell of cordite in the air. Jimmy and Michael were looking a bit pale. It transpired that they had found a stray bullet on the way from school, Jimmy had put it on the gas cooker and they both hid behind the fridge to see what would happen. It went off with a bang and the kitchen was filled with smoke.

Siti liked to cook 'English food,' as she called it. This consisted of rather stodgy cakes and puddings. We preferred it when she cooked Malay dishes for us. She was a dab hand at curries and her chicken rendang was much appreciated. She always got up with the sunrise and came in to cook breakfast for John before he went to work. She cooked usually lumpy porridge followed by bacon and eggs. He once asked if, being a muslim, she minded cooking bacon. Her reply was enlightening. "Siti want job, Siti cook bacon." 2 to 4pm was her siesta time and no one dared to disturb her in the afternoon. Considering she worked from 6am to 6pm unless we were entertaining, when she would stay around until 10pm or later, we thought she deserved her afternoon nap. I often tried to tell her to take more time off. She seemed to have no life outside our little area. I insisted that she had weekends off. Sometimes she would go out and visit relatives but these visits were rare. One morning I came down and she was looking quite ill. It was a bout of 'flu'. I persuaded her to go home and rest. She was worried that I wouldn't be able to manage without her, but eventually I made her see that it was much better for her to rest and get better than to carry on and get worse. Reluctantly she agreed to let the gardener drive her home. We had no idea where she lived when she wasn't in our little granny flat. The next morning there was a knock at the door and a young Malay girl stood there. She was a beautiful girl with honey coloured skin and big brown eyes. "Siti send me." She said. It turned out that she was Siti's daughter. We didn't know that she had a daughter or that she had been married.

When Siti came back I couldn't resist asking her if there were any more children. "One only," she said, "and one *kanak*." I took this to mean that she had a grandchild somewhere. "Where is your husband?" I said, "he go away," she replied fatalistically. In a way I was pleased that at least Siti had a family life of her own.

Life on the married quarters was not without its little dramas One new years eve in 1975 we had all been seeing in the New Year in the Tanglin Officers club. One of our announcers was working in the studios and when he had finished the broadcast, ushering in 1976, we all, in a mildly drunken state, trooped over to the studios to join him for a celebratory drink. Inevitably this turned into a bit of a party and we all staggered back in the early hours. At 4am there was a frantic banging on our door. It was our announcer. "Can I come in, my wife has just tried to kill me." Apparently, she had been waiting at home since midnight for him to finish his shift and had the champagne on ice to celebrate the New Year. We felt guilty. When we had all trooped off to hijack him and bring him to the party we gave no thought to his wife sitting home alone on New Year. The same announcer had a son, Christopher. He grew up to be quite a respectable young man, but at the time we all thought he was weird. If there was a party at the house Chris would sit on the stairs covered in a blanket, watching the proceedings. He had an ongoing battle with their amah, he would go out of his way to annoy her. We could hear her chasing him shouting, "Chrissy, Chrissy, why you so bloody damn bad."

One of our trainee announcers at the time was Sarah Bawden, later to become Sarah Kennedy. After a whirlwind romance, she married Charles Kennedy, a young officer on the garrison. Sarah was very ambitious and gradually she realised that the life of an army wife would destroy her career. Unfortunately, the marriage failed. It takes a lot of sacrifice and dedication to commit to follow the drum. The British military had mainly pulled out of Singapore, but there were a handful of soldiers left, along with Australian and New Zealand regiments. There was a cinema on the camp and, sticking to tradition the national anthem was played at the end of every performance and we, of course, would all stand. After one performance a small group of native Chinese soldiers sitting in the back remained resolutely sitting down as 'God save the Queen' was struck up. This was some kind of protest, an affirmation that Singapore belonged to the Singaporeans. Without saying a word six or seven British squaddies, in unison, slowly inched their way along the rows of seats towards the Chinese lads. Nothing was said, but they stood up very quickly.

On one occasion we found rat droppings in our kitchen. John set a humane trap. It was a wire cage with a trap door that would close when the rat went in to investigate. Sara came rushing in to our bedroom. "Dad, there's a mouse in the trap." We came down to have a look and there was the rat, a fairly large specimen. John took it to the river and threw it in. When Sara came home from school enquiring where it was, John told her he had taken it over the other side of the camp and set it free. A few weeks later at a school open day we were looking through Sara's work books. On the, 'activity, what we did today,' page Sara had written 'Daddy found a rat and took it over to the soldiers quarters'. In the margin the teacher had written one word, 'charming,' followed by a big exclamation mark.

The Singapore climate encourages growth, and so it was with our coconut. One of the children had dropped a coconut behind the cooker and forgotten about it. Within a month we had the beginnings of a small palm tree growing up between the cooker and the wall. When Siti told us that coconut palms can grow up to ten or more feet, we thought it was better to remove it to the garden.

The Hindus and Tamils love their celebrations and Thai Pusam, is one of the more memorable ones. Held in January or February, devotees, mainly Tamils, after a month of prayer and fasting make their way to the temple. Their bodies are pierced with nails and spikes are forced through their cheeks. They drag heavy loads attached to their backs by hooks pierced through their skin. A strange thing is that they appear to feel no pain and there is no blood. Another religious festival is held in July and August. Known as Theemithi, the supplicants, in return for a blessing or a favour from the Goddess Draupadi, will walk barefoot over a bed of glowing coals. This celebration takes place the evening before Divali, the Festival of Light. I witnessed all of these at one time or another, along with many lion dances and a snake charmer.

Occasionally we would take a trip to the Government rest house in Malaysia. It was a little haven situated on one of the islands, Tioman, if I remember correctly. We would drive up over the Straits of Malacca, through Johore Bahru, along the silk road to the island. There was dense jungle most of the way and we could see the monkeys in the trees. We would look at them and they would look back at us. It was illegal to harm the monkeys in Singapore and they knew they were safe. Occasionally, when the soldiers went for jungle warfare training the monkeys would congregate in the trees to watch. The boatman that ferried us to the island was a cool character. He sat in the front steering the boat while smoking marijuana all the way.

I sometimes took the rickety bus to Changi village. There was always a busy market there and makeshift shops lined the road. We could buy anything there, from a key ring with a very rude slogan to a full dinner set of noritake china and everything else in between

Another adventure was a bus trip to the Arab street quarter in downtown Singapore. As well as the usual market stalls and the old ladies sitting on the ground surrounded by live chickens and boxes of uncooked prawns and live crabs, I found the gemstone shops. These were all in one street. At one end were the larger and more expensive shops. The further up the street I went, the poorer it became until at the market end of the street there were makeshift shops under canvas, but they were filled with an unimaginable array of genuine gemstones. I started to collect these stones. Every week I would take the bus and browse all the stalls. I reckoned to buy a gemstone every week. In the end I had a collection which included emeralds, rubies, sapphires, and unusual stones such as tourmaline, black star quartz, jasper and moonstones. These I put in a velvet lined box which I made. I was very proud of this collection. When we eventually moved to Germany I had a pendant made from the emeralds. Some of these stones have disappeared over the years, some I have given to my grandson and most of them I still have.

I had resigned myself to the fact that there were no openings for English nurses in Singapore. The colonial influence was still strong and British ladies didn't work. Instead, I decided to enjoy everything else that was on offer. The social life was excellent and the wives would gather in the afternoons for a game of Mah Jong. I'm afraid I could never be as enthusiastic or aggressive a player as some of the wives. The local SSAFA (soldiers sailors and airman's families association) was staffed by health visitors and social workers. They had a clinic on the married quarters patch. I wandered over there one afternoon to see what was going on and finished up as a volunteer. It wasn't proper paid nursing but I was able to use my experience in several ways, deputising for the health visitor when she was on her visits. A car would be sent to pick me up and I would man the clinic for the occasional afternoon. This was as near as I could get to nursing so it satisfied my need to be doing something useful.

Things changed dramatically in 1975 when Saigon fell to the North Vietnamese. Saigon was the capital of South Vietnam. In April 1975. The People's Army of Vietnam overran Saigon. Prior to that the American families had begun to evacuate the city. Thousands of South Vietnamese citizens were making plans to escape, whether by boat or plane. The military and diplomatic families in Singapore were advised that there could be a mass evacuation of refugees to Singapore. Contingency plans were in place to accommodate these people. Anyone with a spare room was asked to prepare to house these refugees. It was all hands to the pump. I was asked to draw up a list of anyone who was able to help in this way. All the wives were coming up with different ideas, and as is usual with a group of wives anywhere, rivalries began to surface. Everyone wanted a major role. The atmosphere was tense, especially as some of the rumour mongers were perpetrating the 'domino theory' This speculated that as soon as Saigon fell, the other South East Asian nations would fall like a pack of dominoes. This was similar to the situation in Cyprus and I was prompted once again to ask, 'is my life always to be spent in a war zone.'

A chapter on Singapore wouldn't be complete without a mention of Bugis Street in the '70's. This was where the 'Kai Tais,' or 'lady boys' would congregate. When the fleet was in there would be riotous gatherings in the Bugis street area. These Chinese and Malay lady boys were transvestites. There were hundreds of them. At a glance it was impossible to tell if they were male or female. Many is the story of a hapless soldier or sailor who would wine and dine one of these people, only to discover later that the attractive lady he had designs on wasn't all he thought she was.

A well known story is told of a group of sailors from one of the ships who climbed on to the flat roof

of a toilet in Bugis Street and performed a 'Zulu Warrior.' (look it up in Wikipedia!)
http://en.wikipedia.org/wiki/Bugis_Street

There was a high incidence of burglary so most of the houses had bars on the French windows. The burglars would employ a little native boy and cover his body in grease so that he could squeeze through the bars and open the door. The Gurkhas, fearless Nepalese soldiers had a reputation for bravery and were respected by the military as fierce fighting men. There was a saying, 'anyone who says he is not afraid to die is either a liar or a Gurkha.' The story goes that a burglar once attempted to enter the home of a Gurkha soldier. As the felon put his hand through the bars the Gurkha raised his khukri - ceremonial knife - and cut off the hand at the wrist.

Time was marching on and after two years in Singapore we were to be posted to Germany. It was with mixed feelings that I left Singapore. Rudyard Kipling echoes this feeling in his poem 'Mandalay'

If you've heard the east a callin' then you'll never heed naught else

you won't never heed naught else but them spicy
garlic smells

and the sunshine and the palm trees and them
tinkly temple bells.

Chapter 8

Celle and Hohne

Landing at RAF Gutersoh after sixteen hour flight we stepped out into a snow covered landscape. To say it was cold just didn't cut it. It was freezing. We had brought sweaters and warm coats but after two years in the heat of Singapore it was a shock to the system. An army landrover was waiting on the tarmac and we piled in to begin the two hour journey to Celle, near Hannover. It was the coldest journey I have ever experienced. The land rover had no heating and we huddled together to try to keep warm. While I was researching this book I asked Sara what she remembered about Germany. "The landrover was cold." She said. This was twenty years after the event.

We arrived at our new married quarter. What a relief! The heating was on full blast and a welcome pack was on the table. We had bread, milk, tea, biscuits and cereal. This was bliss. Then a knock came at the door. One of the BFBS wives came and introduced herself. She had with her a big dish of shepherds pie and a bottle of wine. We had never had a welcome like this before. Television for the forces was in its infancy. They operated from a mobile truck parked on the camp. Pre recorded tapes of popular programmes and news were sent by plane to Gutersloh. They were collected and rushed to the truck to be transmitted to the troops. In the beginning there were very few programmes except the news, but that grew until eventually we had - wonder of wonders - programmes like Coronation street and Boquet of barbed wire.

The hair raising dash to get the tapes to Celle in time to monitor their content and put them on air involved a lot of ingenuity on behalf of the engineers and presenters. The German winters were so cold that the BFBS truck occasionally froze and the engineer, in most cases John, as he was the youngest, had to lie underneath it in the snow with a hairdryer. The families sitting in comfort in their centrally heated quarters had no idea of the frantic scrabble to get their favourite programmes on air.

In the early days BFBS television had a close working relationship with London Weekend Television and would borrow their announcers and cameramen on a secondment. These very experienced professionals taught our people a lot about television broadcasting. BFBS had had a radio presence for years and everyone knew the ropes, but TV was a different ball game. It involved a new mind set. No longer could a disk jockey sit in front of a microphone in his vest and pants in the summer. He was in vision! It entailed a certain amount of discipline. BFBS personnel were flown back to LWT and BBC in London for regular courses and training sessions. Many of the presenters went on to join the BBC and further their careers. There was Patrick Lunt and Paul Brown, to name just two.

As is usual with expatriates overseas, the social life was lively. There would be dinner parties and mess functions most weeks. Alcohol was cheap, too cheap, some would say and some of the troops filled their windscreen wipers with gin as it was cheaper than antifreeze. We had the occasional publicity visits from UK celebrities One of the more memorable ones was the visit by Tom Baker, or Dr Who. He arrived at Hohne with his entourage. His distinctive scarf and wide brimmed hat, making him instantly recognisable. Tom was a larger than life character, he visited the schools to chat to the children who were spellbound. The army wined and dined him and his team royally. A highlight was the visit to Hohne ranges. The army pulled out all the stops. Tom and his people were treated to live firing displays and tank movements. To cap it all the army arranged a lunch right on the ranges, complete with regimental silver, all under canvas.

At one time there were rumours of prowlers hanging round the quarters and the men were being extra vigilant. It was in the middle of yet another dinner party when the hostess said she could hear footsteps outside. A fair amount of alcohol had been consumed and the guests were ready for a showdown. We all rushed out to find a young German lad on the doorstep. Grabbing him unceremoniously, four of our brave men pinioned his arms and demanded to know what he was doing prowling around married quarters. The poor lad, who spoke no English, pointed across the road to a car belonging to one of our guests. We all looked and saw a plume of smoke emanating from the windows. The interior was full of smoke and there was a glow of fire just beginning. Don, our host, rushed towards the fire. "Stand back everybody, let's get this out." He was brandishing a fire extinguisher from the hall and strode determinedly toward the car. His wife, Susan, a histrionic and voluble lady, was hanging on to his coat tails. "Come back Don, come back, you've a wife and children." Someone had phoned the fire brigade as the wind caught the flames and the car began to burn merrily. By the time the German fire brigade arrived the car was a burnt out wreck. The owner, the unfortunate chap who, in the previous chapter narrowly escaped being murdered by his wife, was preparing to go on holiday the next day and all their passports and luggage went up with the car. To add insult to injury someone suggested that he had arranged it all as an insurance scam. "But why would I burn my own passport?" he asked in a hurt voice.

Another dinner party at the same house caused me some anxiety. The large dining table was placed in a corner and I was seated between the host, a man weighing about eighteen stone and the engineer, another corpulent figure. My back was against the wall, hemming me in. One of the latest 'must have', things on the party circuit in the '70's was a fondue. The fondue set was in the middle of the table. It consisted of an oil filled burner underneath and a bowl of cheese and meat on top. The guests would each have a skewer and would fish the meat out. This was a novelty and we were all in high spirits. Don, again the host, decided that it was burning too slowly and went to fetch some paraffin. His hands were none too steady as he recklessly upended the can. There was a 'whoosh' sound, and flames leapt about a foot into the air. Hemmed in as I was between the two largest men in the room, I had visions of being burned alive. I did the only thing I could. I ducked under the table and escaped among the trousered legs and high heels. The flames eventually died down with no harm done, but from that time onwards I paid a lot of attention to where I sat at parties.

The children had started at yet another school and as Jimmy was now thirteen he was old enough to go to town on the bus with his friends. After one trip he arrived home with a white hamster. "His name is Spiffy," he announced proudly. We placed him in a box while we bought a cage from the pet shop. The whole family had loads of fun watching Spiffy. We bought him a wheel and he would spend hours running on it. He would also swing along from one end of the cage to the other hanging from the bars. One of our more theatrical guests enthused. "That hamster has a tremendous personality."

Matthew was the son of one of the engineers. He was quite a lad. Aged about eight at the time, he discovered a dead carp on the banks of the river. It had been dead quite a while and the smell was horrendous. Nevertheless, young Matthew carted the fish back to married quarters. He went knocking on every door in the street proudly displaying the rotting fish. "Look what I caught." He announced. His dad soon disposed of it

With the children in school I now began to think about work. This time there were no obstacles to my working. I applied for a job at the medical reception centre (MRS) at Hohne, about twenty miles away. There was just one obstacle, I didn't drive. I had toyed with the idea of learning to drive several times over the years but never really got down to it. I had always said 'If I'm motivated I will learn.' What better motivation than a new job? I contacted a military driving instructor from the transport section and he agreed to give me a crash course over three weekends. I gulped when he said 'crash course,' until he explained that it was a course condensed into six days of driving and nothing to do with wrecking a car. The next three weekends were taken up with driving all day and learning the highway code in the evenings. It paid off because three weeks later I was the proud owner of a driving license. It was then that the real learning began. The first day I set out on my own was nervewracking. It got easier though, and soon I was confident enough to apply for the job in Hohne.

Bergen Hohne was my first job in Germany. It was another scary posting. The MRS was an old German building, it was circular in shape with inter connecting doors. As with most older German buildings, it was solidly built with thick walls and sturdy swing doors connecting the wards. At night it was staffed by a nurse and a medical orderly. Being so near to Belsen concentration camp, just a mile or so up the road, it was inevitable that ghostly stories would emerge. By this time in my career I had become more sceptical, and wasn't so easily scared by ghost stories but there were some unexplained phenomena surrounding the roundhouse, as it was known. At about 3am when everything was quiet, my colleague and I would become aware of a drop in temperature, a kind of subtle change in the atmosphere. We would then hear a faint sound as if a trolley was being pushed up the ward. The sound grew nearer and we heard the unmistakable swish of the swing doors. There were six swing doors and the noise grew louder as whatever it was approached us. Then, as quickly as it had appeared, the noise died away. We never actually saw anything, not least because we were glued to the safety of the office. This happened at least twice and many medics and nurses were reluctant to work at the round house at night.

As I lived twenty miles away I needed the car to get to work. Being a very new driver and not yet having the confidence to overtake I would frequently get stuck behind a convoy of tanks on the long road from Hohne to Celle. I formed my opinion of drivers at that time based on my naive experiences. The Germans drove very fast but they were predictable. They took risks but they were controlled risks. The Dutch, however, were unpredictable and impulsive drivers. If ever I found myself behind a car with a Dutch registration I was extra careful. Being a Brit, what they thought of my driving I can only speculate.

The MRS in Hohne was situated on an army barracks not far from Hohne ranges. It doubled as a casualty unit as well as a general surgery with five doctors plus six full time nurses and medics. The sound of heavy artillery from the ranges could be heard frequently. The medics were serving soldiers while the nurses were mostly wives of soldiers and civilians who happened to be qualified nurses. I have frequently been heard to remark that I have never been short of a job whether I wanted one or not. It was not unusual to be called out to an emergency. The phone would ring and the ambulance driver would grab a medic and a nurse. Off we would go, blue lights flashing and sirens blaring. It could be anything from a road accident to a coma. These calls seemed to come in runs, usually some quiet weeks followed by three ambulance runs in a few days. After a quiet run of about a month with nothing except routine, we received a 999 call. A centurion tank - some 20 tons - had gone down an incline and the tank commander, a young captain, had been standing up in the turret at the time. He had very serious head injuries. It was apparent from a distance that there was a skull fracture. His face was grossly out of shape. He was conscious and complaining of severe toothache. We turned on the blue light and siren and sped towards the hospital. Often we never get to know the outcome of these types of accidents. This soldier was eventually discharged from the army on medical grounds and we lost touch but I have often wondered what became of him.

For some unexplainable reason Thursdays were usually a quiet day at the MRS. There were no clinics and the usual run of nursing duties, taking blood, dressings and syringing ears hardly kept us busy. It was usual to enter every patient and their ailment into a report book but occasionally on a Thursday some wag would become bored and a few unprofessional comments would appear in the book. For example, 'private Jones: Complaint: 'says he has a stiff foot but on examination it was found to be only six inches.' This kind of thing was nipped in the bud when the sergeant in charge, a wizened old trooper, reminded us that, "that book is a legal document."

Most new babies were born at the military hospital in Hannover. As it was a journey of about an hour we occasionally had to accompany a mother in an advanced stage of labour. Mrs Davies, the wife of a corporal, had six children and was expecting the seventh. She arrived at the medical centre in the middle of a busy clinic, with contractions every four minutes. Her last delivery had been quick and almost effortless. The duty midwife didn't think she would make it to the hospital. We took her up to one of the wards in the round house and, sure enough, the baby was born half an hour later. A healthy little girl. Mrs Davies was over the moon. We then loaded them both into the ambulance and took them to Hannover. It was just routine, as with any birth outside the hospital, mother and baby needed to be seen and logged in. Mrs Davies was protesting loudly. "I've just had the baby, what do they expect to do at Hannover?" She spent the night there and was discharged the next morning into the care of the health visitors and visiting midwife.

Another ambulance call was for a soldier who had been involved in a road accident. He had been thrown forward and had extensive and deep cuts to his forehead and scalp. One of our civilian doctors, Dr Bannerjee, was on the scene and expertly stitched his forehead. Dr Bannerjee had an interest in plastic surgery and welcomed the chance of a break from routine general practice duties. He put eighteen sutures in the soldier's head before sending him to hospital for X rays. Somehow he managed to blend the sutures into a natural crease in the soldier's forehead. Six months later there was hardly a scar.

Another call out we had was to a road accident on the camp. No one was really hurt but the car was badly damaged. We arrived at the scene where a small crowd had gathered. The driver's wife was loudly haranguing her husband and calling him an idiot. The front of the car was stoved in and a thin stream of liquid was trickling towards the crowd. I couldn't tell if it was water from the radiator or leaking fuel. Just as I was attempting to move the onlookers back a few yards for safety reasons, I watched, horrified as a soldier threw the butt of a lighted cigarette on to the ground. Things moved in slow motion. They say this happens in dangerous situations but I had never experienced it before. Slowly I watched the cigarette arc through the air to land right in the path of the liquid. It was water. Never have I felt so relieved.

One of our corporal medics prided himself on being a crack shot with a rifle. He was a member of the gun club on camp. He had served in Aden and had shot for the army at Bisley. The role of an army medic is essentially a non combatant role but Eddie took great delight in telling us how he had shot a few Arabs in Aden. I didn't know whether to believe him or not. Certainly he was a crack shot with an elastic band and chewed paper pellets. I have seen him shoot a fly out of the air. "You need to anticipate where he will be in the next five seconds and aim your missile there," he told me. I must confess, it must have taken a lot of experience to plot the trajectory of a fly.

Many of our civilian drivers at Hohne were displaced Poles who had drifted to Germany after the war. They were a mixed bunch, but all quite friendly and obliging. The soldiers overseas had certain perks such as an allowance of duty free petrol and cigarettes.

A lively black market had sprung up between the soldiers and the drivers. The currency was NAAFI cigarettes. Occasionally civilian visitors were flown out to Hohne on liaison visits and it was an opportunity for them to stock up on duty free whisky and vodka. One such visitor, a Ministry of Defence civil servant, came to the camp. He was being shown around by the commanding officer. He had been to the NAAFI for his duty free whisky and had it with him in a plastic bag. This man left the bag in one of the offices while he was inspecting the facilities. On returning to the office the bag was nowhere to be seen. We searched everywhere. It had disappeared. Eddie, the corporal said, "leave it with me sir," and strode off in the direction of the civilian driver's quarters. He came back some ten minutes later clutching the whisky. Nothing was said and the civil servant went on his way happy.

Whenever we had visitors to Hohne, one of the places they all wanted to visit was Belsen, the site of the concentration camp. To say it was grim would be an understatement. It was bleak. No trees grew and no birds sang. When the British liberated Belsen in 1945 the conditions there sickened them. 50,000 people died at Belsen. Jews, Czechs, Poles, homosexuals, Roma gypsies, Christians, not to mention 20,000 Russians. Belsen was a holding camp, there were no gas chambers. Most of the deaths were from starvation and typhus, which was running rampant. Also tuberculosis and dysentery. After the war the concentration camp was rased to the ground using tanks and flame throwers. Thousands of bodies were buried in mass graves and covered with quick lime. No trees or greenery could survive because of the lime in the soil, therefore there were no birds to sing. Anne Frank died there in 1945, aged fifteen. Even today the brooding silence hits you as you go through the gate.

Chapter9

Werl and Hamm

All too soon our posting at Celle came to an end. This time it wasn't back to England, as we had expected, but to Werl in the Soest region of North Rhine Westphalia. The nearest large town was Dortmund. Most of our colleagues lived in married quarters on Werl station. Owing to a shortage of living accommodation we were housed in Hamm, some ten miles away from the camp. We lived in a block of German occupied flats. At first I was disappointed not to be on the camp with everyone else, but the children learned to speak German fluently and made friends among the locals. Windsor school, a forces boarding and day school was just up the road and most of the teachers lived nearby. About this time Sara had started to get romanticised ideas about boarding. She read all the children's books and was fascinated by the idea of midnight feasts in the dorm and all the fun the boarders seemed to enjoy. We knew by now that we would be travelling for the foreseeable future, and that they needed continuity of education. I was very much against the idea at first. I could see the sense in the argument but she was my little girl and I was reluctant to let her go. We started to research girl's boarding schools in the UK and finally decided on Red Maid's school in Bristol. We took Sara to have a look and she seemed enthusiastic. It had a very good record academically and the girls seemed happy enough. Also, I had trained as a nurse in Bristol and knew the city well. So it was that in the September term she became a boarder. It was the biggest sacrifice I have ever had to make. I came back home and cried for a week. Not so Sara. She settled in quickly and it was only after a few terms when the novelty had worn off that we had a few complaints. "The ratatouille is too greasy. I'm not going to wear hockey boots. The biology teacher doesn't like me."

Every half term and school holidays all the boarders would come home on the 'Lollipop special', flying to Gutersloh. The younger children, up to the age of thirteen had labels on their luggage and were known as UNMINS. - unaccompanied minors. The airline staff would look after them during the flight and see them safely on and off the plane. Sara was most indignant at being labelled an UNMIN. Jimmy had been a boarder at a boys school in Taunton, Somerset for a while but when he reached sixteen he wanted to come back and go to sixth form college at Windsor school. It was good to have at least one of my children with me. There was a constant stream of Jim's mates at our house, all teenagers at a loose end. For his seventeenth birthday we bought him a moped. He would whizz around the school area trying to do wheelies while I watched with my heart in my mouth. His love of motorbikes never diminished and he owned one until recently when a wife and four children interfered with his youth. The original moped went for about a year, when it started to splutter and cut out. It turned out that some of the German lads in the flats had urinated in his petrol tank. There was nearly a turf war.

Living in a mainly German environment we became more aware of the rules and regulations. This was demonstrated one Sunday. John was washing the car when a little red headed four year old strode up. "*Das ist verboten.*" She said sternly. It was not done to wash ones car or peg washing out on a Sunday. Even the little children knew that. Who did this English interloper think he was! John just grinned and said. "It's alright, I am the mad English." The little tot accepted this and wandered away.

Once again I became restless. I was a nurse, for goodness sake! and I needed to work. A vacancy was advertised at the medical centre in Werl. I went for the interview ready to take my place against the competition. There was no competition. The medical officer, when the interview was finished said. "I'm giving you the job, you are the only applicant." This did nothing for my confidence. I would have liked some competition. I just got the feeling that the job was mine by default. It was not the best way to start. The regiment at the time was a Scottish one, The Black watch, based at Albuera Barracks. An old established regiment with a proud history and tradition. Their unique uniform with the tartan trews made them stand out. The 'Jocks' as they were known, are a warlike people by nature. They enjoy a fight. This was borne out every Saturday night in the bars around Werl and Hamm. We received frequent ambulance calls, though the Royal Military Police had many more. No matter how much of a melee they had been involved in over the weekend, these soldiers always appeared on parade immaculate on Monday morning.

Accommodation on Werl barracks consisted of blocks of flats. One of these was near the medical centre building. A sergeant and his family lived there. The wife, Mrs Mcgregor, was a large woman, some twenty stone or more. She suffered with spinal problems and occasionally her back would go into spasm. She would call out the ambulance and the medics would attempt to manhandle her huge bulk down the stairs More often than not they couldn't manage it and the Medical officer, who didn't do home visits, would have to go up and sort her out.

One more unusual patient I remember was sergeant Hammond. He arrived at the medical centre one evening accompanied by his wife. As he walked in through the door it was obvious that something was wrong. His whole body was leaning to the left and his face appeared paralysed down one side. This had come on gradually over a period of hours. Assuming it was a stroke, I called the ambulance to take him directly to the military hospital. I was surprised when, the next day he appeared at the medical centre perfectly straight, with no sign of the previous night's trauma. They had run all the tests and had come to the conclusion that the cause of his problem was a severe migraine attack. There had been no headache and no visual disturbance.

After some time at Werl a vacancy had come up for a school nurse at the boy's boarding school in Hamm. I had always wanted to try my hand at school nursing and the vacancy was right on my doorstep. Saying goodbye to Werl medical centre, which had never had the same appeal as the busy one at Hohne, I started on what would become one of the most rewarding periods of my career.

The senior nurse at Hamm at the time was Madge. She was a divorcee who had lived a chequered life since parting from her husband. A stint as a nurse on board a cruise liner as well as spending some years as a matron in a retirement home for elderly theatrical people in Northolt was part of her CV. Madge was a character. Now in her 60's, she held court as queen of the officer's mess. There was talk of a relationship with one of the civilian administrative staff, a man of similar vintage. But Madge had the wanderlust. She moved from Hamm in the late 1970's and the last I heard she had taken a live in position as matron at a retirement home near Hampshire. It was run by a flamboyant gay couple. I kept in touch with her for several years and the last I heard she was in an on/off relationship with a widower somewhere in the home counties.

Another colleague was Marie, who grew to be a lifelong friend. We both had teenage children at the time and the school job was convenient for the school holidays. Marie would occasionally arrive at my door with a bottle of wine and we would put the world to rights. She was studying for an open university degree at the time and I admired her dedication. Eventually she gained a BA, and we were all justifiably proud of her.

The medical centre was never very busy so there was plenty of opportunities to chat to the boys. It was usually the same dozen or so pupils that we saw most of the time. As with any boarding school there was the problem of home sickness among the younger ones. A lot of them just needed to know there was someone who would listen to their problems. A school nurse's job is as much pastoral as medical. The older boys were usually 'army brats' - the common name for forces children. They were street wise, they had travelled and were well used to disruption. Forces children are endlessly adaptable and learn to be self reliant at an early age. There was a window on the ground floor of the school building with a faulty catch. It was well known among the sixth form boarders who would creep in after lights out. The following morning they would appear in the medical centre with a hangover.

One of the funnier episodes was the story of a lad called Phillip. He turned up at sick bay with a perfectly circular bruise in the middle of his forehead. It took just one look and I knew what he had done. "OK," I said, "Where is the sucker?" he looked innocent. "What sucker? "He asked." The rubber sucker that shoots from toy guns and sticks to windows," I replied. "Oh, that sucker," he grinned. "How did you know?" "I haven't been a nurse for 20 years and not come across that kind of bruise." I said. Another time he came with a badly bruised knuckle. By this time I knew him well, he was one of my regulars. "If you must punch the wall, please try to use some padding." I said in what I thought was a severe voice.

The school doctor would visit every other week. He was old school and a bit theatrical. He specialised in sports injuries and with a school population of around 200, he had plenty of scope to practice his expertise. 'Exercise, tubigrip knee supports and ice packs' was his mantra. He had little patience for something as mundane as a sore throat or a cough. "Ask sister for a paracetamol," was his solution to many problems. He loved his sports injuries, though.

In the summer holidays the teachers who lived on the camp would organise events such as barbecues and dances. These were open to everyone. One memorable evening somebody thought up the idea of an auction. We would all bring along unwanted items and they would be auctioned. The proceeds would go towards new sports equipment for the pupils. This was well attended and wine was flowing to aid the bidding. I had my eye on a black and white television set for the sick bay. Waiting impatiently until this lot came up, I joined in the bidding. Quite soon the first bidders dropped out and there were just two of us left. The bidding was going higher as the other lady was bidding against me every time. The teacher who was acting as auctioneer began to look worried. We were in danger of bidding for more than the value of the set. I glanced across at the other bidder. It suddenly dawned on me that this was no longer about the TV set. It was a military versus civilian competition. There is always a degree of rivalry between the military and civilians on an army camp. The perception - quite wrongly - is that the 'civvies' have all the perks. Having been on both sides of the fence, I understood this. The other bidder had a steely glint in her eye and a determined expression. She wasn't going to give up. I did the only thing I could. I withdrew. If sick bay wanted a TV we would club together and buy one.

Forces Television was growing and expanding. It was decided to move the unit down to Joint Headquarters, Rheindahlen. Another move. This time it was much easier to pack everything up. By now I was used to travelling light. The BFBS station prepared to move en masse to Rheindahlen. I had heard rumours that the post for a UK based civilian sister at Kent school was being disbanded and there would be a vacancy for a nursing sister from the local population. Naturally, I applied. Thus began another adventure.

Chapter 10
Knuckles, Bones and Fangs.

By this time I had gained a fair amount of experience, both in medical centre nursing and school nursing. The interview went well and I emerged as the new sick bay sister at Chatham House, the boarding wing of Kent school.

The sick bay was situated at the end of a long corridor. At one end was the boarding house accommodation for the girls and the teacher's flats, and at the other end was the sick bay. It consisted of two wards, each containing three beds, and a sitting and bathroom for the duty sister. We worked an unusual shift pattern, twentyfour hours on duty and fortyeight hours off. There were two other nurses so that one of us would be on duty at all times. It was a shift pattern that suited me as there was ample free time while putting in full time hours. An adjoining block was for the boy's accommodation. We had a clinic at 8am before school started, and another at 6pm before supper. Any child with a temperature or other illness would spend the day in the ward. We found that on Thursdays when the pupils had double maths, our morning clinic would be full.

As with the sick bay at Hamm, there were the usual regulars. Some of these we saw most days. I suppose any medical practice anywhere in the world will have its share of the 'worried well'. Out of the hundreds of children who passed through Kent School, inevitably there are some who stand out. One such was Fred, a cheeky thirteen year old. He was popular with everyone. The housemaster tells the story of when the boys were in the common room, he noticed Fred absentmindedly scratching his nether regions. The teacher said, "don't play with yourself in public, Fred." Later that evening when he went to put the lights out in the dormitory, a little voice piped up. "Can I play with myself now Sir?"

Another more alarming incident sticks in my memory. It was about 3am when there was a frantic knocking on my door. Grabbing my dressing gown I rushed out. Two boys were standing there. Quick, sister, Alan Donovan is having a brain storm." I rushed down the corridor, not knowing what I would find.

Young Alan, fast asleep, was smashing the exit door with his shoe. He stood there oblivious to everything around him, repeatedly banging the door. The glass had shattered in tiny pieces. Avoiding the glass, I gently walked up to him, put my arm around his shoulders and walked him back to sick bay. He didn't even wake up. Next morning he had no recollection of what he had done. I called out the duty housemaster and left him to deal with the back door and somehow make the building secure again.

Most teachers are given nicknames by the pupils, but I didn't think it applied to the nurses. I was wrong. One of my colleagues suffered from arthritis and her hands were badly deformed. She earned the nickname 'Knuckles'. The other one was quite tall and thin, so the children called her 'Bones'. I have always had irregular front teeth, so I was known as 'Fangs' Of course, it was supposed that we didn't know about this. I can't speak for my colleagues, but I knew. One of the drivers told me.

Another of the boys was always very pale, combined with hair so fair as to be almost translucent. He earned the nickname 'Casper.' There was a children's comic at the time featuring a character called 'Casper the friendly ghost'

When one is dealing with teenagers there is always the question of pregnancy and contraception. It was a Sunday afternoon when one of the teachers came over for a chat. Apparently two of the older girls had approached her regarding their friend, who thought she might be pregnant. She asked me if I would call the girl in and see if there was any truth in the rumour. I knew I would have to handle this delicately, and, quite frankly, I didn't know where to start. I discussed this with my colleagues whose overwhelming response was that they were glad I was the one to deal with the problem, not either of them. So much for solidarity.

Fortunately for me I didn't have to call the girl in. She appeared in sick bay in tears, asking to talk to a nurse. I invited her in to my sitting room and, over a cup of tea, she admitted that her period was six weeks late. On further questioning she admitted to having sexual intercourse just once with her boy friend. Her form mistress wanted me to send her to the medical centre immediately and was all prepared to inform the girl's mother. I, on the other hand, was minded to wait another two weeks and see what happened. I had done a pregnancy test that proved negative, so I felt it was sensible to wait and see. The Sixth form was preparing for their 'A' level exams, and it was a fairly tense time for all of them. Often this kind of tension can interfere with one's body clock. This, combined with the negative pregnancy test reinforced my decision to wait and see. I now had to deal with the housemistress. She, being in 'loco parentis,' was worried. She felt responsible for the welfare of her pupils. She didn't agree with my 'wait and see,' policy. I was older and more experienced. I explained the situation from my point of view. How would the girl feel if we contacted the medical centre and her parents if it turned out to be a false alarm? Not only would the girl be shamed and embarrassed, but the parents trust in the school would be compromised. I said that another two weeks would make little difference anyway. Reluctantly she conceded. The next two weeks were an anxious time for us all, not to mention the girl herself. She popped into the sick bay most days, just for support and reassurance. Two weeks later we were vindicated. She came to tell us that the panic was over, nature had taken its course. I used the opportunity to have a talk about contraception. The housemistress came that evening, much relieved that she had allowed herself to be persuaded to wait.

All of a sudden, on April 2nd, 1982, we found ourselves at war. This came virtually out of the blue. No one had expected it. Argentina had invaded the Falkland Islands, claiming that these barren windswept islands belonged to them. For 150 years the Falkland Islands had been British. The then prime minister, Margaret Thatcher, was having none of that! Mrs Thatcher possessed more bulldog spirit than the whole of her cabinet together. With little or no hesitation and close consultation with the heads of the armed forces, it was decided that we would fight back. To Mrs Thatcher it was the only option.

The boarders at school were old enough to realise the danger this situation presented. With the added problems of being away from home, it was a tense time for all of them. A team of counsellors came to the school and the pupils were invited to come along to sick bay and chat to them. There was the civilian youth counsellor, who we all knew, then the psychiatric social worker as well as two health visitors that SSAFA sent along. In the event, the only professionals the children wanted to talk to were the ones they knew. The youth counsellor, along with the nurses, were kept busy. We all listened anxiously to the radio every morning and the mood for the day was determined by the report on the news. Euphoria if it was good, and worry if it was bad.

On the 2nd April the Argentines invaded the Falklands. On the 5th April a task force was deployed from the UK. The 25th April saw South Georgia taken by the Royal marines. The 4th May was a bad day. HMS Sheffield was hit by an Exocet missile and lost and a British jump jet plane was shot down over Goose Green. The SAS (special air service) saw casualties when one of their helicopters was hit. On the 14th June we were all euphoric as we heard the news that the British flag was raised over Port Stanley. On 16th June the Argentinian President, General Galtieri resigned. It had been a traumatic and tense two months. The feeling of relief was palpable.

The fall out from the war was to be felt for many months. Post traumatic stress wasn't recognised at the time. The soldiers who had been to the Falklands and seen war at first hand would carry the images for the rest of their lives. Many of them had developed strategies to deal with it but there were some who were permanently damaged by what they had seen and done. At the time the welfare services were having to deal with an unusual number of marital problems among the families. The Falklands war acted as a catalyst. It was decided that some form of marriage guidance was needed. An open letter was sent to all the military families in Germany asking for volunteers to apply for selection for Relate training This came at a time when I was actively looking for something more challenging than school nursing. I thoroughly enjoyed my job but I felt there was more I could do. The letter about Relate training was exactly what I had been subconsciously looking for.

I applied, along with about thirty others from the families on Rheindahlen. We attended a month long series of selection interviews, group sessions and individual assessments. It was narrowed down to seven and we started our training. The training was ongoing over a period of two years, with a further year to become accredited. Herbert Gray College in Rugby was the venue for the UK part of the course. The seven of us were flown to the college every three months for intensive group training sessions. In between we had more sessions in Germany. After the first six months we started actual counselling with couples on the camp. There were weekly discussion groups with an experienced Relate trained counsellor who acted as our mentor. There we could raise issues that had arisen from the clients we had seen. It was an open discussion between the seven new counsellors and our mentor. We didn't use names in these discussions. Before Relate training I would have said there was not much new that I hadn't already learned. How wrong I was! The training was intense and it was only in the following years that gradually we all became aware of a new dimension. It's difficult to put into words the subtle changes in the group. I became more aware of atmospheres, what was said and what was meant. Our mentor called it 'hearing the music behind the words'. This training helped me immensely in my school nursing as well as personal growth.

After eighteen months of sessions at the college and actual counselling we were invited to join a psycho sexual counselling course. It was felt by the powers that be, that all seven of us were ready to take it to the next stage. We all trooped to the airport in a state of high excitement. Not only was it a trip back to UK, but psycho sexual counselling was something new and intriguing. By this time the group had gelled and we were all firm friends. We probably knew more about each other than our families did. One of the objects of the course was to familiarise ourselves with the sexual content of our counselling and to feel free to talk openly to our clients about sexual matters if that is where their problems lay. We were shown fairly graphic videos and heard tapes of sexual counselling sessions from couples who had agreed to be taped. These discussion sessions with other groups from all over England were designed to break down barriers and help us to be able to speak freely and without embarrassment. After an exhilarating week the seven of us caught the train back to the airport. We were all on a high. It had been a stimulating week and we were discussing everything that we had seen and learned. It was only when we noticed that a few heads were turning in our direction and we slowly realised that we weren't in a group session now. We were back in the real world. The heady atmosphere of the last week had to be modified somewhat.

One interesting episode concerns Sally, a chatty fourteen year old, who had been coming to the clinic every morning for a week. Her complaints were a bit vague and non specific though I got the feeling that there was something worrying her. She stayed behind one morning after the other pupils had left for the school bus. I said, "Come on Sally, you'll miss the bus." Bursting into tears, Sally told me she had been having the same nightmare for months. There was someone standing over the bed looking at her. "It's so real, I can actually see her." We talked at length about this. "She was wearing a white coat, and I wake up terrified. I'm sweating and my heart is pounding as if I've run a race." I told her she could come to sick bay whenever she needed to talk about this. During the following weeks we saw her several times, though the nightmares didn't go away. The breakthrough came some six weeks later. I noticed that she had scars on her neck and arms, obviously from scalding. At the next session I turned the conversation round and asked her what had happened. When Sally was tiny a pan of boiling water had fallen on her, resulting in a long and painful spell in hospital. Over a couple more sessions we explored a scenario where a little girl, in intense pain from burns, would wake up and see a nurse standing by her bed. To a tiny child, this memory, combined with the pain, would have imprinted herself on her mind. Added to this was the fact that she was away from the comfort of her home, as she had been all those years ago. Miraculously, when we had fully explored these feelings, the nightmares stopped. I heard years later that she had qualified as a psychotherapist. It's strange the things that influence the paths we take.

I had an old radio in my room in the sick bay and at one of the clinics, Nigel, a sixth former, showed particular interest in it. "Wow! where did you get that antique radio from?" He enquired. I was amazed. I could remember buying that radio some years ago. If that was an antique, what was I? The same lad came to sick bay for a chat. He was telling me a story about one of his fellow students, a girl in the same year as him. Reading between the lines, when he had mentioned her name for the sixth time, I deduced that Nigel was smitten. Ah, teenage first love and teenage angst! I couldn't place the girl, she was not a regular visitor to sick bay. "You know who I mean," he said earnestly. He had been chatting for half an hour and I had work to do. Maybe I was a bit flippant, but I replied, "I can't place her, all teenagers look the same to me." It was the wrong thing to say. He glared at me and walked out.

About that time Chatham the kitten made his appearance. Around midnight I was woken up by a very loud sound. In my half asleep state I couldn't identify it. It was somewhere between a baby's cry and a screech. Jumping out of bed, I looked out of the window. There was a tiny kitten in the grounds of the boarding house. It was hard to believe that all this noise was coming from him. I rushed around to the back door hoping to get into the garden to rescue him. It was locked. The only way for me to get into the garden was through the sick bay window. Standing on a chair, I climbed through. It was a ground floor window so I could manage fairly well. The kitten was tiny, his eyes were barely open. I put him in my dressing gown pocket and climbed back through the window. He was shivering. I fed him a few drops of milk from my finger, which he sucked eagerly, put him in my sheepskin slipper to keep him warm and he settled down to sleep. The next morning I put him in a cardboard box, loaded him in my car and drove home.

Sara happened to be home from boarding school and she took charge. She bought a doll's feeding bottle from the NAAFI toy department and went to a pet shop in Rheindahlen to enquire about what milk to feed him with. We called him Chatham, after Chatham House where I found him. All went well for a couple of weeks, then one morning he wouldn't take his milk, he just lay in his box, listless. I thought if we watched him and kept him warm he would perk up, but Sara was having none of that. It had to be a visit to the vet. Off we went to the vet in Rheindahlen village. It was just as well we did because Chatham had cat flu. The vet was very kind but said the kitten, being so young and having been abandoned, was unlikely to survive. He agreed to give him a vaccination though he told us it was probably too late. Chatham surprised us all. In a matter of days he was fully recovered, he regarded us as his family and would lick our hands as if he was washing us. He followed Sara everywhere. The problem was, being a feral cat, when he got a bit older he would spray everywhere to mark his territory. Our bedroom was considered fair game, and we had to vacate it and open the windows for three days before we could get rid of the tomcat smell. While we were both at work we would leave the bathroom window open so that he could come and go as he pleased. At 3.30 each day the day school children would come home from school and Chatham used to climb out of the window to play with them. He thought he was human. The kids got to expect this and would wait outside the house for him.

One awful day I received a call in work from our neighbour. Chatham had been hit by a car as he was crossing the road to join the children. I couldn't leave sick bay so John went home. The kitten was badly injured so John took him to the vet. On the way he was licking John's hand as if to reassure him. The vet said to leave Chatham with him and he would see what could be done. As it turned out the injuries were too severe and poor little Chatham died. I have never had a cat since.

Chapter 11

Itinerant Nursing in UK

We knew it was likely that our next posting would be back to UK. It would either be Chalfont St Giles or Paddington. The priority was to buy a house within commuting distance of both these places.

As often happens in these situations, fate intervened. Mr Chang, our Chinese tenant moved with his family up to London so the house was empty again. When we went to put it in the hands of an estate agent we discovered that Mr Chang's two sons had dug and planted the garden. They had laid one half to lawn and the other half was given over to rows of potatoes, lettuce and carrots. Given the trauma I had suffered in trying to cultivate it when we first moved in, I was delighted. It was a selling point, too.

We started house hunting in the Home Counties area. This was difficult as we were still in Germany. Every post brought brochures advertising houses, some of which were way beyond our budget. We decided we must have a plan. When we had narrowed the list down to six houses. John booked leave and we drove over to

UK. This was the beginning of a long nine months of searching. Some of the houses we saw were quite run down, others were outrageously expensive. It seemed to us that house prices were escalating every month. It was a difficult few months. Eventually John went over on his own for a week. It was in term time so I had to work. He phoned me at work, "I think I've found the right place," he sounded excited. It turned out to be a mock Tudor semi in Ruislip, Middlesex. It was twenty minutes from Eastcote tube station with a regular bus service outside our door. The garden was planted with roses and when I flew over to have a look, they were in bloom. This house ticked all the boxes so, when all the formalities were completed we took possession. Later that year, as we expected, John was posted to Paddington. It was ten tears since we had last lived in England.

After three months settling in, I began to get restless. I wanted to work. After the relative freedom of school nursing and casualty work, I didn't fancy the regimented regime of hospital work. What to do next? The answer came from an unexpected source. At a party I was chatting to a colleague of John's. She had been a nurse but had given it up for a nine to five job some years ago. "Why don't you try industrial nursing?" She asked me. This was a totally new field to me. I would never have thought of it. An agency had opened up in central London and they specialised in supplying nurses to larger department stores and factories. At that time the emphasis was very much centred on health and safety at work. Many of the larger firms had their own medical centres. These were usually staffed by one full time nurse, so there was a demand for agency nurses to fill in for sickness and holidays. This agency had more or less cornered the market for supplying industrial nurses. I went for the interview. By this time my CV was growing and my experience with the military stood me in good stead. I raked out my old uniform. Fortunately it still fitted although I had to let the belt out a few inches. The list of clients read like a page from 'Who's who.' There was a week at Harrods, a month at Robert Maxwell's printing works in Watford, De Beers, the diamond merchant, London Weekend Television, The BBC at White City, Marks and Spencer, the Rolls Royce factory. I could go on, but I've forgotten many of them. Suffice it to say, the agency had the monopoly of high profile businesses around London.

All of these had a small surgery in the workplace. The work was never strenuous. It involved arranging appointments and medicals for the works doctor, usually a GP who would do contract work on a private basis for the employer. The unions were powerful at that time and health care was part of the package they had negotiated with the management. I would be on the scene in case of accidents at work and see to minor ailments such as headaches and nosebleeds.

Harrods was very much involved with the welfare of their workers. They employed a staff counsellor to iron out potential problems while they were still manageable. The car bomb that had devastated Harrods in December 1983 had left a legacy in its wake. Whereas none of the Harrods employees had been killed, six other people in the vicinity of the car lost their lives. Three were policemen who had arrived at the scene in answer to a warning phone call, and the other three were innocent civilians. The nurse who was on duty at the time described the scene to me. "We witnessed everything in slow motion," she told me.

"People were screaming and running for the doors. I went into auto pilot," she said. "We were trying to keep everyone calm, but we had no idea if there was another bomb hidden in the store. The police, fire services and ambulances blocked the street, there was a general air of disbelief. The weeks that followed were tense and difficult. Several of our staff were afraid to come into work, some suffered delayed shock reactions such as flashbacks and panic attacks. It was after this that a counsellor joined the staff."

My month at Robert Maxwell's Mirror group in Watford was a real insight as to how a factory worked. I could see vast conveyor belts bringing the printed newspapers and magazines rolling off the press. It was a massive building complex with departments for printing, typesetting and assembling newspapers. Everyone was conscious that they were working to a deadline. The news must be out there, whatever the problems. The stress level was high. There was a steady stream of patients at the medical room, mainly with stress related problems. Being in a stressful environment had an effect on me and I was always glad to relax on the drive home with my tapes and favourite tracks. I would pour a large gin and tonic when I got home and that would put things right.

De Beers diamond merchants was a revelation. I was thrilled to get this assignment. I had visions of being able to see magnificent diamonds, all sparkling before my eyes. Nothing could be further from the truth. The medical room was set apart from the main body of the building. I was escorted there by a security guard and given a name tag. Diamonds, before they are sorted into industrial or jewellery grade, look like any other granite stones you would see on the road. One of the patients came to the medical room with a painful shoulder. As she took her coat off a tiny stone fell out. It looked like a piece of grit. I was quite unprepared for her reaction. "Oh my gosh!" she said, "I'll be in trouble if anyone sees that." Apparently it was an industrial diamond. The staff were regularly searched on leaving the building and security was tight. The diamonds that were not pure enough for jewellery would be used to make cutting and grinding implements for factories. Nothing was wasted. Round about lunchtime the phone rang. It was someone enquiring what I would like for my lunch. I had expected to go to the works canteen, as was the usual practice. Not so at De Beers! A chef arrived complete with white overalls and carrying a covered serving platter. On the plate were three little birds and an assortment of vegetables in separate serving dishes. Apparently these were quails. They looked so sweet on the plate that I couldn't bring myself to eat them. That was not all. For dessert they served a perfect miniature pavlova. How the other half live!

Another place where security was tight was Wembley Stadium. I did one shift there. Once again a security guard led me to the medical room. I did not see a single patient. The guard told me that, unless there was a big sporting event taking place, the nurse was employed mainly to pacify the unions. It would be most unusual to be called upon to do any work. I wondered if the resident nurse had died of boredom.

The Rolls Royce factory in Watford was another security conscious assignment. It was a fascinating place. The foreman took me on a tour of the building and I was allowed to see these magnificent cars being assembled. The thing that struck me most was the pride everyone showed in their work. Each person was at great pains to explain his or her part in the manufacturing process. As with De Beers, there were very few patients. I have a theory that the number of sick employees bears a direct relationship to the job satisfaction of the individual. Some factories are happy ones and some have a high level of discontent. Rolls Royce was a good one. The building was massive and stretched over thousands of yards. There were twists and turns, large workshops and small specialised units. The medical room was somewhere near the exit, down a corridor. About 5 pm I heard a bell, not thinking much about it I went on sorting paperwork. Ten minutes later the phone rang. It was the foreman. "Aren't you going home?" He enquired. I thought my shift ended at six. "The bell went ten minutes ago," he said. I packed up what I was doing and made my way to where I thought the exit was. The factory appeared deserted. I must have taken a wrong turn. Try as I might, I couldn't find the exit. I wandered round for about fifteen minutes when the security guard approached me. "Are you lost?" He asked with a grin. At that point I was very near to tears. "We've been watching you on the security camera for the last ten minutes," he said. My sense of direction isn't very good at the best of times, but this was the last straw. The next day when I arrived to start another shift there he handed me a ball of string. "What's this for?" I asked. "You tie it to the exit and follow it to the medical room and you won't get lost." "Hah! Very funny," I said. I hoped I sounded suitably sarcastic.

The Glaxo pharmaceutical complex was yet another on my list. Out on the road towards Greenford in Middlesex, it was a large imposing building. They were very much involved in research and the medical room had a well stocked reference library. As well as normal nursing duties the team of nurses there were encouraged to keep up with all the new innovations in medicine. It was quite a high powered environment and the nurses were very much part of the team. I worked there for a month via the agency. It was a good example of forward thinking and innovation.

As a contrast to the Glaxo building there was a brewery near Hounslow. The smell of hops was overpowering at first but soon I didn't notice it. The factory was noisy although the medical room was away from the main body of the building. The company doctor would visit twice a year and the duty nurse would arrange medicals for the staff. Blood was taken to measure liver function and blood pressure was measured as routine. Being a brewery, there were two or three known alcoholics on the workforce. The nurse would keep an eye on their health and provide counselling when the need arose. The staff were allowed a ration of cheap alcohol as one of the perks of the job. As with most of the factories, there was a security guard on the gate. The nurses had a visitor's pass which had to be handed in after a shift. Passing through the gate I stopped to hand in my pass. Jumping out of the car I took it over to the guard. Calamity! I had slammed the car door with the keys inside and the engine running. It was a very old ford fiesta. I tried rattling the windows and pulling on the door but it wouldn't budge. The guard suggested covering the exhaust so that the engine would stall. That didn't work either. After fifteen wasted minutes in which we tried everything the guard and I could think of, I was resigned to breaking the window. A crowd had gathered by then and I heard someone say, "send for Cliff." I didn't know who Cliff was, but evidently the others did. He arrived in a couple of minutes. "Right." He said. "What's the problem here?" It was obvious what the problem was, but I humoured him. "Okay nurse, turn your back," he commanded. Reluctantly I did as I was told, then, in about a minute and a half a miracle happened. The door opened and the engine stopped running. What a relief! When I got home I told John about it. All he said was, "Ask him how to hot wire it as well".

The BBC television centre at White City in West London was one of my last assignments. Their medical room was at Wood lane centre. If I had expected to see some famous faces I was destined to be disappointed. In the two weeks I worked there no one from the television appeared. Every day there would be a small crowd of fans waiting around the gates as I drove in. They would peer through the car window and when they saw it was only me, they would shrug their shoulders as if to say, 'That's nobody famous'. I wondered what it must be like to be a genuine celebrity.

After a year of this type of work, the old wanderlust kicked in. I wanted a change. I craved real patients and continuity. Answering an advert for a practice nurse in nearby Harrow Weald, I embarked on the next phase. The practice employed four doctors, one nurse, a receptionist and the practice manager. Eva, the practice manager, had been in the job for over twenty years. She had guided the practice through all the changes that the NHS had imposed, and kept a close eye on how the practice was run. We all deferred to her. Eva had something of a reputation amongst the local surgeries. She had an encyclopaedic grasp of all the protocol and minutiae of running a practice. Her pet hate was keeping the patient's notes in order. There were approximately two thousand patients on the books. Before the days of computerised records the patient's notes were kept in buff folders. Some of the patients had been with the practice for over twenty years and their folders had become a bit dog eared. The notes were kept in alphabetical order in a series of shelves along the wall. The secretary would set out the folders for the next day's appointments the evening before. Inevitably, some of the notes couldn't be found. The first place we looked was in the doctor's surgeries. Doctors aren't taught about filing in medical school! If this failed we would have to do a search of all the records. Woe betide the person who had filed something in the wrong place. The newest recruit to the practice was Fiona, a GP on her first proper job after training. Eva intimidated her so much that after misfiling two or three sets of notes, causing us to literally strip the shelves, Fiona wouldn't go near the office. She used to drive a beat up volkswagen with a bent wire coat hanger as a radio aerial. She had the makings of an excellent GP, kind with both adults and children, Fiona would allow time to listen to their problems, so much so that she often ran late. Occasionally she would call me into the surgery to confirm her diagnosis of a rash. In my time as a school nurse I had seen measles, mumps, rubella (German measles) chicken pox, nappy rash, prickly heat, viral rashes that disappeared after twentyfour hours and in one case, meningitis. I prided myself on being able to identify most childhood rashes. I blotted my copybook with Eva on one memorable occasion. The practice used my experience as a marriage guidance counsellor on the odd occasion. One of our patients had been having a traumatic time dealing with retirement.

Instead of a busy working environment this lady suddenly found herself at home all day. To make matters worse, her husband had retired at the same time. Instead of them both having their own careers and personal space, they found themselves too much in each others company. It was a difficult time and they were both trying to adjust to it. "He has taken over the kitchen," she moaned "And I can't even do the weekly shop without his input. And the TV remote control, don't get me started on that subject." There was very little I could give in the way of advice. This was new to me. Most of my previous counselling experience had been with much younger military families where the problems were different. I sensed that the marriage was basically strong and that she just wanted to let off steam. She talked non stop for over an hour and on leaving said she felt better for the space to talk. I reassured her and told her that I was here any time she needed to unburden herself. I had taken her case notes with me to have a read through before the session and familiarise myself with her background. The next day was my day off and when I returned to work on the Wednesday it was to a scene of chaos. The shelf full of patient's notes was emptied on to the desk and Eva was incandescent. Where was Mrs Fulton's notes? They had searched everywhere. I had a sudden feeling of dread. I knew exactly where those notes were. Now, should I own up and admit that I had left them in the counselling room or should I quietly return them to the shelf? The decision was made for me. Eva looked at me and said accusingly, "you were the last person to see Mrs Fulton. I don't suppose you took her notes?" I had to admit it was me. I was persona non grata for the rest of the day.

As the practice grew we began to think about extra clinics. It was decided that there should be a family planning clinic attached to the surgery. Although I had given family planning advice on a regular basis in Cyprus and Germany, I had not got, 'the certificate.' This, in the 1980's was the buzz word. Health care was expanding month by month and new avenues were opening up for nurses to specialise. It was an exciting time. I was sent on a three month course at Northwick Park near Harrow. This course was structured so that the participants spent some time in the classroom, interspersed with secondments to various clinics. There was a week at the clinic for sexually transmitted diseases at the Central Middlesex Hospital, (the clap clinic) as it was known. There we were introduced to the range of drugs in current use and learned to identify various organisms through a microscope. It was a busy clinic with a minimum of one hundred patients seen each week. Their ailments ranged from syphilis, which was rare since penicillin, right through the range to simple candida infection (though it wasn't so simple if you happened to be the patient.) We learned about the morning after pill, which was quite new at the time, and became familiar with the full range of contraceptive pills and devices on the market. The next session was a week at a family planning clinic in Ruislip. We were taught how to fit diaphragms (Dutch caps), and practise taking cervical smears.

A highlight of the course was the visit to the London Rubber Company, - the johnny factory. We went in groups of six. By this time we had all become friends and were all looking forward to the visit. We were met by an eager young man in a suit. I'm afraid he was a bit intimidated by six voluble nurses. He took us on a tour of the building, introducing us to various departments. It was a surprise to learn that they also made marigold rubber gloves there. We were shown the process by which liquid rubber was made into contraceptives, and told about the various types of condom that was manufactured there. I hadn't realised there was such a range and variety. The next phase caused us a great deal of hilarity. It was the area where they tested the products for durability. Behind a glass case was a great iron machine with a central column. A condom was placed on this and it commenced to move and vibrate. The object was to see if the condom was strong enough for normal use and that it had no holes. Apparently they tested ten out of every batch. Our supervisor said to us. "Now girls, no witty remarks, they have heard them all before." At the end of the visit we were each given a goody bag. It contained a pair of rubber gloves, a variety of different condoms, about ten in number, and leaflets detailing the work of the London Rubber Company. I took my goody bag home and the kids, who were grown up by then, were fascinated, especially when I told them about the machine. Over the next three months or so all the condoms slowly disappeared. I didn't question my son or daughter too closely.

Another month was spent at a family planning clinic at Stonebridge park. This was very much a hands on experience. It was where we put our newly learned skills into practise. Stonebridge park was a run down area in direct contrast to our experience at Harrow. While I was there the doctor's car was broken into by teenagers looking for drugs. The consultant was a charismatic figure. She was a tall woman with an intimidating presence. On my first day there she cornered me. "Ah, nurse, now what have you learned on this course?" She boomed. I was able to detail most of the work and she questioned me minutely on the finer points. My experience in Cyprus, combined with the recent placements, enabled me to acquit myself reasonably well. I left with my family planning certificate. Another string to my bow.

Two years seemed to be my limit in a job before I got itchy feet. Maybe it was the itinerant lifestyle I had married into but whatever the reason, I started looking around for another challenge. It came in the form of a conversation I had with an old colleague. Along with health and safety at work, preventive medicine seemed to be the way to go. Many commercial outfits had jumped on the bandwagon. They aimed to provide a mobile screening service to any firm that was willing to pay. Occupational Health International (OHI) was just starting up. They were looking for experienced screening nurses to staff their mobile van. The idea was that they would travel round UK with a team of nurses, a driver and a radiographer. The van was equipped with facilities for a full range of health care plus an X ray room for mammograms. This sounded good to me, especially as the contract stipulated that I would work one week on and one week off. We were a mixed bunch as we set off on our first assignment. It was a small engineering firm outside London. In the mornings we screened the male employees, measuring cholesterol, blood pressure and giving general health advice. A health assessment was printed out on the computer - a new toy for me. This was then given to the patient along with advice about smoking, alcohol and diet. There was some suspicion at first amongst the male employees. They wanted to know if a copy of their results were sent to the management. We were able to reassure them that the overall statistics were sent to the management to enable them to identify potential problems and to put in place strategies to avoid them. The individual assessments were entirely confidential. It was the turn of the ladies in the afternoon. The same comprehensive questionnaire was shown to them as well as cervical cytology and mammograms.

The radiographer was getting over a divorce, and she had taken the job as a means of escape. Her children were grown up and the job was the first step on her journey to full independence. The other nurses had a similar background to me. They had both travelled, one as a WREN, and one as an air hostess. We had a lot in common. The only difference was that I was the only one with a husband. They expressed surprise that I would take on a job where I was away from home so much. I replied that it was only one week at a time, the pay was good and my husband frequently spent days away with his job. Where we could, we would co-ordinate our work schedule. After six months I began to sense a change was imminent. The orders had stopped coming in and we were spending more time at the headquarters in Buckinghamshire. The writing was on the wall and it wasn't long before the firm closed down. A casualty of the increased competition.

The next adventure was with a similar firm, but this time with a much more professional approach and a solid backing. American Medical International (AMI) was the same set up as OHI, but with years of experience behind them and a sound financial backing. The work pattern was the same, though this time there were two teams of nurses. One covered the London area and worked mainly in the medical rooms of the firms and factories. The other team worked from another mobile van, usually parked in the car park of the venue to be screened. I started off with the van. As before, we had three nurses, Linda, Laura and me. There was a radiographer, Mandy, and a driver, David. We stayed in hotels while we were working. All day long we saw a stream of patients and in the evenings we had dinner and a few glasses of wine in the hotel. It was a cosy little set up. One of the nurses, Laura, had a phobia about cleanliness. She would virtually strip her room in the hotel looking for anything that shouldn't be there. It was not unusual for her to change her room more than twice until she was satisfied there were no germs. Linda, the other nurse, was a happy go lucky girl. She would have slept in a tent if the need arose. Linda also liked a few glasses of wine, she was fun to be with.

The first six months of mobile work on the van was exciting, but after a while, when I would wake up in a hotel bedroom and wonder where I was this week, the novelty began to wear off. Our supervisor, an older, very experienced nurse manager, probably sensed this. One Monday morning she called us it to the office near Regents Park. "Six months is long enough in one venue," she said. "I'm swapping the teams around." This was a shock. Our team had gelled and we all got on well. Laura was to join the in house medical team, Linda was to alternate every other week with me, as she was ready to cut down her hours. I was to join the team that covered the London area. At least it would mean no more hotels, or so I thought. I also would be at home every evening. My new team mates were Freda and Felicity, known by everyone as Flick. My first assignment with the new team was with a financial firm in Hammersmith. It was a massive glass walled building. Security was tight and we were given passes to clip on our dresses. The medical room was seven floors up with a view all over London. It was equipped like a modern private hospital. Every facility was there, and everything looked brand new. There appeared to be a very strong hierarchy in this place. The managers all came at a specified time by appointment. The traders came next, they were much younger and a lively crowd, mainly ex public schoolboys with one or two barrow boys to add to the mix. They wore an unofficial uniform of red braces under a striped blazer. Very much further down the chain were the secretaries and receptionists. The overall topic of conversation seemed to be money. I suppose it was financial institution, after all. I was left wondering if they had any other values beyond trading the next million.

Our next job was at Marks and Spencers in Harrow. They had a reputation for looking after their staff. This was somewhat dented in later years when they outsourced their manufacturing base to India in order to save money. We were allowed to eat in the

Marks and Spencer's canteen where we had our pick of their food hall. This was one of the perks I enjoyed. There was some confusion as to where we would sit in the canteen. There seemed to be designated places and we didn't want to sit in the wrong one. Where did nurses come in the pecking order? Eventually we found an empty table and sat down. There were several curious stares, but nobody moved us on. Afterwards, one of the staff said they thought we were store detectives.

When we changed teams I thought it was the end of living in hotels and travelling, but there were a few more trips to come. I had been with the new team for three months when we were asked if we would mind covering Scotland on a temporary basis. So it was that we flew to Glasgow for a week, covering the Post Office employees. The following month it was Edinburgh, then Perth. I enjoyed these sessions once I had learned to understand the Glaswegian dialect. Our working day finished at three thirty, so there was time to explore the shops. This time we stayed at an upmarket B&B. The owner and his wife were a colourful couple. Tanya, the wife wore a flowing kaftan and beads, and Jim, the husband would play the bagpipes in the evening in full highland dress. We would gather round while sipping scotch and soda.

Chapter 12

Germany Revisited.

We had been five years in UK. It was time to move on. We eagerly awaited the next posting. Would it be somewhere warm, Gibraltar maybe? This was not to be. It turned out to be Rheindahlen again. I wasn't disappointed, I knew Germany and I had picked up enough of the language to feel confident. There was a slight problem initially with housing. Apparently there were no married quarters available for a month. John went on ahead while I waited in UK for the phone call to join him. During that month I made arrangements to let our house in Ruislip. Strangely enough it was to another Chinese man. We had had such a good experience with the previous Chinese tenant, that I had no qualms about this one. When the phone call came I was all ready for the move. John drove over from Germany and picked me up and so began yet another adventure.

The story I am about to relate may stretch the reader's imagination, but it is entirely true. Our married quarter had four spacious bedrooms plus an attic and a cellar. It had been standing empty for three months. I must confess that I wondered why this quarter had been empty when I had waited a month in UK to be housed. The first month was spent settling in. It was only after six weeks in the quarter that strange things started to happen. We were preparing to go out one evening and I wanted to wear a favourite topaz ring. This ring had been on the mantelpiece for two or three days so I knew where to find it. All dressed up, I went to find the ring. It wasn't there. After searching everywhere it still couldn't be found. Reluctantly I chose another ring from my jewellery box and forgot about it. Two days later I was sitting on the bed in the spare room sorting out the ironing. I heard a, 'plop,' sound behind me, and there, on the bed, was the ring. A few of John's colleagues asked me how I was settling in to the quarter. I thought nothing of it, supposing it was just a polite enquiry. When the fourth or fifth person asked me the same question I thought it a bit odd. A week or so later I came downstairs one morning to find a small emerald on the dining room table. I immediately checked my jewellery box. There were a few rings I had picked up in Singapore, one of them had three tiny emeralds. It was intact. So where had the emerald come from? I put it in an ash tray to investigate later on. When I went to look at it the next day it had vanished. Yet another time John was in the bath when there was a splash behind him and a piece of chocolate plopped into the water. "Aha! Caught you," he grinned. I had been dieting and he thought I was having a sneaky bar of chocolate. I was most indignant. I hadn't touched chocolate for three weeks (a great sacrifice on my part.) So where did the chocolate come from? On four or five occasions the door bell would ring on the dot of 6pm. There would be nobody there. Sara, our daughter was out on a visit. On her first morning she stood at the top of the stairs in her pyjamas. "Mam, somebody has died in this house," she said. We hadn't mentioned the strange happenings, as we hadn't wanted to frighten her. "Don't be silly," said John. A little too quickly, I thought. Occasionally I would find a small pool of water on the table. There was no sign of a leak anywhere, and the table was in the middle of the room away from any of the taps. Strangely enough, there was never a creepy feeling to the house, it was just a normal married quarter. The house was in immaculate condition when we moved in, all except the downstairs cloakroom. There were what looked like rust stains on the floor behind the behind the unit. One day, I put on a pair of rubber gloves and bleach, determined to get rid of them. As I scrubbed, the stains came away easily and there were little bits of gravel wedged behind the pipe. The reason for this wouldn't become clear until I started work in the medical centre some three months later.

One of the first things we did was to look for a car for me. If I was going to get a job I would need transport. I needed a little run around. Not a high powered thing, just something that wouldn't be too expensive to run and not too big. After several visits to dealers and garages I settled on a Volkswagen beetle. It was a vivid orange colour - fashionable at the time. I drove it round the camp a few times to get used to the feel of it. John went to work and, thrilled with my new purchase, I decided to take it for a run. I drove into the village, did some shopping and headed for home. Stopping on the way to show it to a friend, I parked expertly. When I returned to the car I had to reverse out of the parking space. That was when I encountered the problem. Where was reverse? I had no idea. Every time I put it in gear it inched forward a few feet. I was terrified of hitting the car in front. There was no more room to manoeuvre. Eventually I did the only thing I could think of. I phoned John in work. The conversation went something like this. Him. "You see the little diagram in front of the gear stick," Me. "Yes." Him. "See the numbers on it," Me. "Yes." Him. "See the little 'R'," Me "Oh yes." Him. "That's reverse." Me, "I did that and it didn't work." Him. "Did you press the gear lever down before moving it?" Me, "I didn't know I had to." Him. "Go back and try again." Me. "I can't, I'm afraid it will go forward again." Him, exasperated. "OK, stay where you are, I'll be over in about ten minutes." My knight in shining armour arrived ten minutes later and reversed out for me. Then he drove me to a patch of waste ground. "Now try reversing again, there's nothing to hit." That's how I learned to reverse. In my defence, I must say that the car I had been driving in UK had a different right hand drive set up.

I went to the medical centre to see if there were any vacancies for nurses. There were none at that time but they took my CV. Two months later I received a phone call. Could I come for an interview. Three other girls were interviewed at the same time. One had just qualified as a nurse, the other had six months to go before she was due to be posted, so I reckoned the only real competition was the third girl. She was about the same age as me and had a similar amount of experience. I had not long arrived on the camp. They probably thought I would be around the longest, but whatever influenced their decision, I got the job. It was shift work. 8pm till 8am on the first day, the third day, 8am till 8 pm, then nights again over the weekend. It averaged out at thirtysix hours a week.

The day shift was much the same as it had been in Cyprus. Four nurses manned the treatment room and dealt with a stream of patients and doctor's requests. As the medical centre was near the NAAFI it was always busy, mainly with minor ailments. The night shift could be quiet or very busy, especially on a Saturday night. A doctor was on call and a single nurse on duty. The door was always locked at night so the patients would have to ring the emergency bell. Often, if it was a genuine emergency we would get a phone call to alert us. I learned from experience that when the bell rang and there was no advance warning it was unlikely to be life threatening. Some of the more memorable incidents concerned a teenage girl, Carol, who was a regular visitor to the medical centre. The bell rang at about midnight. It was Carol. She had a tea towel wrapped round her arm. "I've cut myself." She said. There were four or five superficial cuts on her arm. I asked her how it had happened. She said that she was stretching to reach the kettle and the knife rack was in the way. This didn't make sense to me. Surely the knives would have been stacked with the blades pointing downwards into the block. I dressed the wounds and gently questioned her further. She stuck to her story. It was obvious to me that she had been hacking at her wrists. I had a word with the doctor and the social worker the next morning and they agreed to keep an eye on her.

Another time the emergency bell rang late at night. I opened the door and a young lad fell in. He was about thirteen or fourteen years old. "Help me," was all he said. When I got him into the treatment room he was barely conscious, though I could see no sign of injury. "I've taken twenty panadol," he whispered before he slipped into unconsciousness. Preparing an emetic, I phoned the doctor who said. "Take him straight to hospital." I called out the duty medic and woke the ambulance driver. RAF Hospital at Wegberg was less than fifteen minutes away and they sped off on a blue light. That was the beginning of a busy night. Within ten minutes the bell went again. This time it was two drunken soldiers who had been in a fight. They were escorted by the military police. One of them had a broken nose, this was obvious at a glance. The other had deep cuts to his face from a broken beer bottle. I patched them up as best I could, advising them to come to the surgery tomorrow morning. They went off to spend the night in custody. The first soldier had his nose set at the hospital the next day. No sooner had they left than a young mother brought her baby with croup. Many of the army wives were very young, away from their families for the first time and with a new baby to care for. Often the husband was away on duty. They relied heavily on the medical centre.

In August 1990, Iraq invaded Kuwait, triggering the first Gulf War. The Americans called it, 'Operation Desert Storm'. To the British contingent it was known as 'Operation Granby'. Once more I was destined to be working in an army medical centre when the troops were preparing to go and fight. We had long queues of soldiers at the vaccination clinics. Rumours circulated that the Iraqi's used chemical warfare and vaccines against anthrax were hastily shipped in. An early form of satellite navigation was popular at the time, especially as it was known to be used by the SAS. It was a Magellan global positioning device. Within weeks the American PX, and the NAAFI had stocked them. It became one of the, 'must have's,' among the soldiers. All leisure activities were suspended and the troops were on almost permanent standby. The effect on the wives and families was evidenced by the extra work load at the medical centre. It was a tense time and everyone was on edge. The stress related illnesses multiplied.

The rumours flying around did nothing to alleviate their fears. Tales of atrocities began to circulate among the troops. A particularly nasty one was how the Iraqis treated their prisoners. British soldiers were issued with what came to be known a 'goolie letter.' It was written in Arabic and English, and basically, it stated that this was a British soldier, and if the Iraqi's didn't castrate him, Her Majesty's Government would give them a sum of money as a reward. It is well known that such a letter was issued to troops in the World War 2. Whether the soldiers in Rheindahlen had one is open to debate. My nursing colleague at the time tells me her husband was issued with one but personally, I never saw it. The insurance sharks began circling the barracks, charging exorbitant life insurance premiums. They offered millions of pounds in compensation for soldier's families if the husband was killed in action.

Thankfully, the Gulf war didn't last long. In February 1991 it was all over. The Iraqi army were driven out. A heavy price had been paid with the loss of 47 British lives, 294 American as well as French and other coalition soldiers. The political repercussions rambled on. A common remark by returning soldiers was that they had been in more danger from American friendly fire than Iraqi weapons. The hidden cost of the war in mental health and post traumatic stress disorder was not immediately recognised. The break up of marriages, due in part to the fact that the men carried around images and trauma in their minds that they couldn't discuss with their wives and families was only slowly revealing itself.

Meanwhile, I had settled into our married quarter and immersed myself in the life of the camp. While chatting to the medic on night duty the conversation turned to the emergency calls he had attended. I asked him what he thought was his worst call out. He thought for a while then said, "It was over in the quarters near the NAAFi, a man had committed suicide. He had shot himself in the head in the downstairs cloakroom. It was pretty gruesome, I can tell you!" Suddenly all the hairs on the back of my neck prickled. I knew what he was going to say next though I didn't dare ask the question. "It was one of the houses in Lewes walk." He continued. I had a terrifying recollection of trying to remove the stains in the cloak room and the little bits of gravel. Obviously, it wasn't gravel, but bone fragments. It was just as well that I didn't know at the time what I was dealing with. Everything fell into place, the reason everyone kept asking me how I was settling in to the quarter, and why there was a delay before we could move in. John had known about it but hadn't said anything as he didn't want to upset me. As I have already stated, there was no sinister feeling to the quarter despite the strange happenings, and once I had got over the shock, life went on as normal.

The new doctor in charge of the medical centre decided we needed a higher profile and he asked me to write an article about health care for the station magazine. It appeared in the next issue and I was asked to contribute on a monthly basis. This was a new venture and I was pleased to give it a go. Having no experience whatsoever of typewriting, I wrote in longhand on paper initially and the secretary typed it up for me. Eventually I bought a word processor and learned to do it myself. Round about 1990 the emphasis was very much on health and safety and preventive medicine. Computers were just beginning to be used widely and many new initiatives were appearing monthly. One of these was the, 'Look after your Heart,' course. This was a six month course leading to a healthcare qualification. I enrolled on the course with a colleague and together we ran classes and groups from the camp. We were asked to give talks at the wives club and various other organisations. With shift work and courses in the evenings, I was beginning to feel the pressure. I wanted a quiet life. About that time, the deputy headmistress of Chatham House, the boarding wing of the school, approached me. There was a vacancy for a senior nurse coming up, and would I be interested. I thought about it for a while, weighing up the advantages. The offer of a job that I loved, plus the bonus of school holidays, proved irresistible. This had come at just the right time. So it was that I joined the boarding house for the second time. In the school holidays I did the occasional shift at the medical centre as holiday or sick replacement, so I had a foot in both camps.

Kevin, one of the boarders was the kind of lad everyone remembered. Although he wasn't ill he would appear regularly in the sick bay for a chat. He would perch on the edge of the couch and chat about anything and everything. His ginger hair was gelled into a spike and in the evenings he wore a single ear ring. This wasn't allowed in school hours, but as soon as he was on the school bus, in went the ear ring. One day he appeared at my door. "I'm well ill, sister." He croaked. Indeed, he looked terrible. I took his temperature, it was 38 though he was shivering. This was the beginning of the, 'big flu epidemic'. The next day there was a long queue at my morning clinic and by the evening Kevin had six other companions in sick bay. This continued for the next three days when the numbers reached thirtytwo. The deputy head came to ask what we should do. The sick bay only had capacity for twelve children at most. We admitted the worst ones but the children who were recovering had to stay in the dormitories in the daytime. This presented a problem for the in house staff. The matron, whose role was to be in charge of the pupil's welfare apart from their health, made the point that she was not medically trained and didn't consider it a part of her remit to look after children in the daytime. I could sympathise with this as, when there are more than six children all throwing up, it presents a problem.

The school holidays were due to start within two weeks and the head wondered if it would be better to close the boarding house down early and send them all home. This sounded the most sensible course of action.

I agreed with her and the administrative staff started the process of ordering buses for the mass evacuation Parents were contacted, and all of this went fairly well. We breathed a collective sigh of relief. Arrangements were made for the whole boarding house to be thoroughly cleaned in preparation for the new term. The next day I received a phone call from the medical centre. Could I pop in and have a chat with the senior medical officer. He was very courteous and diplomatic, but I was made aware that, in order to do something as important as to virtually close down a school, procedures had to be put in place. He, as medical officer in chief of the garrison, was ultimately responsible. What added insult to injury was the fact that all the teachers were employed as civilian staff and, as such, were regarded by the majority of serving soldiers as at best, different. Maybe I had been naive, but I learned a lesson in local politics and diplomacy.

Living and working closely with the military with their frequent deployments to dangerous places we are saddened, but not surprised by news of death or injury. It was brought closer to home one cold day in June 1994. My co worker in the, 'Look after your heart' project received the terrible news that her husband had been killed in a helicopter crash over the Mull of Kintyre when returning from a conference in Inverness. All twentyfive passengers and four crew were killed, including MI5 operatives, British Army intelligence experts and Royal Ulster Constabulary. It was the largest peacetime tragedy the RAF had suffered. The shock waves were felt all over the military community.

Post traumatic stress disorder - PTSD- was beginning to be recognised by the military, and I was offered the opportunity to attend a course at Church House, Lubbecke. It was called a Clinical Incident Debriefing Course. There were about thirty people attending, ranging from soldiers, social workers, nurses and health visitors. It was a lively course lasting from Thursday evening to Monday morning. The lecturers were a mixture of military and civilian psychiatrists and psychiatric social workers. We were shown videos of interviews, and personal accounts of soldiers returning from Iraq. This course was invaluable experience for my counselling sessions. I emerged with a much greater understanding of PTSD, plus another certificate to add to my growing collection.

Meanwhile my job as a school nurse kept my feet on the ground. I had a regular clientele of about eight regular customers, including Kevin, the lad I mentioned earlier. One day he came looking a bit guilty. A pop group at the time wore safety pins in their ears instead of ear rings and Kevin had been trying to fit a safety pin where his ear ring should have been. Teenage boys have only a mild acquaintance with hygiene, and it had become infected. His earlobe was red and swollen, it looked quite sore. I cleaned it with eusol and he came back every day for a week to have it redone. It healed well, but the hole had scarred over. About a month later he came again asking me if I would put the safety pin through his ear. Needless to say, I sent him on his way.

On another occasion my doorbell rang late at night. There were two boys and a girl escorting another boy who was wandering around with a vacant expression. His pupils were dilated much more than was normal. The other kids swore he hadn't taken drugs and there was no evidence of alcohol. I decided to play safe and send him to the medical centre to be assessed. I had a word with the young doctor on duty. "His pupils are quite dilated considering the amount of light." I said. "Hmm, yes," was her reply. His friends had walked him round for an hour before bringing him to sick bay. Despite intense questioning they maintained that he had not been taking drugs of any kind. Knowing that he would have been expelled immediately if this proved to be the case, I could see their point of view. The doctor took a blood sample and sent him back with the instruction to keep him in sick bay overnight and in future to keep a close eye on him.

The boys and girl's dormitories were in two adjoining buildings. These were old prefabricated buildings from pre war times. They had been updated and modernised for use as boarding houses. The doors were locked at 11pm and the buildings were secured for the night. What no one had foreseen was the fact that, with a bit of ingenuity, the boys could climb out of a window and access the roof. From there they could jump over to the roof of the girl's block. This was not only totally forbidden, but extremely dangerous. This practice came to light one night when the housemistress was doing her rounds at midnight. She heard a thumping sound and looked up toward the skylight. Two shadows flitted past her vision and disappeared. She immediately alerted the housemaster in the boy's block. He went to investigate and found the open window. The housemistress did an inspection of the girl's dormitory and found another window on the latch. Everyone appeared to be asleep. She secured the window and waited. After two or three minutes the boys appeared on the roof. Finding the window closed they made their way back. On reaching their block they climbed back through the window, only to find the housemaster waiting. That was the end of that little game

At 11pm two boys appeared at sick bay. One was supporting the other who was obviously very drunk. I thought I had better admit him for the night to let him sleep it off. At 3am I heard him vomiting. I was afraid that, in his drunken state he would inhale the vomit and choke himself so I sat in his room all night to make sure he was safe. It was a very sad and sorry Kevin who got on the school bus the next morning. I hoped he had learned his lesson, but I wouldn't hold my breath. Another of the boys (the girls were much less trouble) came to sick bay very agitated. He looked grey and was unsteady on his feet. His mates said that he had been inhaling the contents of an aerosol of deodorant to see what it felt like. As I wasn't sure of the effects of this I sent him to the medical centre. They kept him overnight to observe him. There were no serious side effects so he was sent back to school and an interview with the headmaster.

I had been at Chatham House for three years. It was time for another move. This time it was Herford in North Rhine Westphalia. Once again we packed up and followed the drum.

Chapter 13

Herford and Bad Oenhausen

Our married quarter was in Bad Oenhausen, one of several married quarters scattered around Herford. It was eight miles from the camp and the drive to work in the mornings was spectacular. In the spring and summer the gardens were full of flowers. In the autumn the gold and russet colours of the trees were magical, and the winter landscape was miles and miles of snowcovered hills whichever way I looked. Most of our friends from Rheindahlen lived in the area and we would have frequent parties and barbeques. I had developed an interest in spinning while I was at Rheindahlen. There was an old German carpenter who made wooden spinning wheels to the exact specifications of the antique ones used in past centuries. I bought one of these and set about finding a farmer who would sell me a fleece. Fortunately the cellars in the married quarters were large and accommodating. There was plenty of room to wash and dry the sheep's wool. A whole fleece was heavy and bulky and saturated with lanolin. It was marvellous for softening my hands but inconvenient to collect and sort into grades of wool. Another girl I met at Herford was also interested in spinning and she told me about a wool factory just out of town. It was an Alladin's cave. We saw massive great bins containing all grades and colours of fleece. The natural colours were the ones I liked best. They had cream, apricot, brown, black and the rare black and white Jacob's fleece. They also had a large selection of dyed fleece of every conceivable colour. I spent countless hours spinning, washing, winding and drying wool. I started to knit. I hadn't knitted since I was thirteen. Starting off with a scarf, I became more ambitious until, eventually I knitted a sweater for Sara. Surprisingly, she wore it. She usually turned her nose up at anything that was home made. My masterpiece was a brown and cream sweater that I made from a pattern in a magazine. The design on the front was a kind of landscape. I was very proud of it. It went everywhere as we travelled. Recently my grand daughter unearthed it from the back of the wardrobe and wore it proudly.

As well as spinning I had developed an interest in airbrush painting. I had always enjoyed painting and drawing, though over the years there hadn't been much time for hobbies. I really threw myself into this, and one Christmas John bought me an air compressor. This, combined with a new airbrush opened up a whole new field for me. I even held a small exhibition of paintings on the camp. The natural progression from this was to make frames for my paintings. Germans are creative and inventive people. There were numerous craft shops in Bad Oenhausen. It was a Spa town and people came from all over the region for, 'The Kur.' This was a three week long session where they had intensive therapy, such as mud baths, exercise, cold showers (Ugh!) and long walks in the surrounding countryside. Many Germans I got to know would say that they were exhausted by the kur, and would need a holiday to recover.

The craft and DIY shops sold lengths of wood cut into patterns to make frames. These came in two metre lengths and could be cut into shape. It was a family joke that for the next birthday I received a black and decker workbench and a mitre saw. I would cut the wood to the size I wanted, and paint the resulting frame in colours to match and blend in with my pictures. If anyone needed me I could be found in the cellar surrounded either by dripping wool or wood shavings.

Bad Oenhausen was a little haven away from the bustle of Herford town. In the summer it attracted thousands of visitors. it was not unusual to see staid German hausfraus stepping off the train in their tweeds and brogues, only to see these same ladies the next day parading in the park in scanty summer dresses and short skirts. These ladies left their inhibitions behind at the railway station. Bad Oenhausen was that kind of town. It was also renowned as a centre for heart surgery and many medical conditions. The spa water was widely believed to have healing qualities due to the minerals it contained. In the centre of the town was a sculpture. It was known as the 'piggy fountain,' and depicted a farmer surrounded by half a dozen bronze pigs. The story behind it was that in previous generations, a farmer couldn't sell his pigs at market because they had developed a skin condition. By chance, while driving them back from the market, his cart overturned and they fell in the river. From that day, so rumour has it, the skin condition was miraculously cured. This led to the discovery of spa water and the growth of the town. The statue commemorates this farmer. The largest craft shop in the town was owned by a man with dyed black hair and colourful clothes. We all thought he was a gigolo. He would flirt outrageously with the middle aged German ladies and they would blush and simper like teenagers.

Our nearest neighbours, Mark and Heather, had a large garden, so somebody suggested they should have a garden gnome. At the bottom of the road there was a shop selling all manner of ceramic figures, from grotesque gargoyles to almost life size garden gnomes. Somebody bought a gnome for them. He was about as tall as a child and took pride of pace on their lawn. One night, after a drunken party, they awoke to find the gnome missing. A ransom note was stuck to a nearby tree. "Give us 100 euros or the gnome gets it," was the menacing message. From that day on, he disappeared and reappeared on a regular basis. I think, in the end, the frost got him.

Once more I began to think about getting a job. The only opening was the medical centre on Herford camp. They were advertising for a senior sister so I applied. Again it was shift work involving a mixture of night and day work. Army medical centres are much the same all over the world and I fitted in seamlessly. We had a team of ten nurses covering twentyfour hours. There were six army medics, a sergeant and a staff sergeant. We had six doctors, two receptionists and a medical secretary. The midwife and health visitor were also based at the medical centre. The senior medical officer at the time was fairly young, I suspected it was his first senior appointment. He was never seen without his laptop, he carried it around like a baby. We used to joke that it was his security blanket. He had an interest in alternative medicine and was experimenting with acupuncture. He bought a set of acupuncture needles on the internet. One of our regular patients, a young woman with chronic back pain, had tried every kind of therapy and drug regime, but nothing gave her any relief for more than a few days. She agreed to try acupuncture. Tony, the young doctor, asked the receptionist to book three appointment slots so that he could treat Mrs Beynon. She got up on the couch and Tony proceeded to insert the needles into various pressure points then told her to relax for a few minutes. Just at that moment a woman rushed in with a child who was gasping. She said that he had just been stung in the neck but she didn't know whether it was a bee or hornet. Tony was the only doctor on duty at the time and this was an emergency. He came out and prescribed piriton then waited to see if it was going to be effective. The child appeared quite drowsy after a few minutes and Tony thought it might be the effects of the piriton. At last the little lad began to perk up and we all breathed a sigh of relief. At that moment the staff sergeant drifted in. "Do you know there's a patient in your surgery with her kit off?" was his remark. "Oh shit!" Tony gasped and went rushing back to his room. We never did find out if the acupuncture was effective but Mrs Beynon remained a frequent visitor to the treatment room.

There was an attempt to streamline the day to day working of the medical centre, it was all to be computerised. To this end we were all sent on a computer course. The younger nurses took to it like a duck to water, but the older ones, that is, the health visitor and me, did not. I struggled. For my generation there was an, 'on' button, and an, 'off' button and that was all that was needed. We couldn't get our heads around the complexity of passwords and computer commands. Even today I rely on John and the grandchildren for the difficult bits, though writing a book has greatly increased my knowledge.

I thought when we moved to Herford that I would no longer be involved in the military's deployments in dangerous places. How wrong could I be! In 1995, after the Bosnian peace agreement a multinational force was set up to enforce this agreement. Some sixty thousand troops from different NATO countries were deployed to Bosnia to act as a barrier between the Serbs and the Croats. It must be stressed that this was a fragile peace. There were still skirmishes breaking out all over the region. Between three and six million landmines had been laid during the hostilities. While it was no longer a conventional war situation, it was still a dangerous posting. Once again the medical centre was over run with soldiers updating their vaccinations and our medics were getting ready to fly out. Our Staff

Sergeant, a veteran with service in Cyprus, Aden, Northern Ireland behind him, was actually looking forward to the posting. Chatting one afternoon, he was regaling us with war stories. "I always knew I would come away with five medals." He said. "Bosnia will be the last." After the troops had left for Bosnia the camp appeared deserted. Many of the wives had gone back to UK while their husbands were away.

It was now thirty years since we had begun travelling. It was time to think about retirement. A posting to the London area had convinced us that we needed a bolt hole away from the congestion and bustle of a big city. We started looking for a weekend retreat. I was in Cardiff on holiday when I walked into a small craft shop. There was a display of paintings by an artist I hadn't heard of but the evocative images of Carreg Samson and chromlechs captivated me. The moody purples and misty grey colours spoke to me. It was a print, but I had to have the original of this painting. The artist, Stan Rosenthal, had recently moved to Saint Davids in Pembrokeshire. The next time we were home on leave I went to Pembrokeshire in search of the original painting. I met the artist and his lovely partner, Nikki, who is now his wife. The studio was full of Stan's colourful works. I was captivated. Also, I fell in love with the area. This was where I wanted our holiday cottage to be. From then on, every time we were home from Germany we drove down to Pembrokeshire in search of our holiday home. Over a period of a year we searched, we must have seen hundreds of properties. There were rural farm cottages with huge ingle nook fireplaces, rambling run down houses that had charm but required a lot of work. Houses beside rivers with water mills. Then, suddenly, we saw the one. We both knew at once. It was an upside down house, meaning that the living accommodation was upstairs and the bedrooms were downstairs. The view from the living room was spectacular. The Preseli hills could be clearly seen and Carn Llidi, a prehistoric mound, was shrouded in mist. As far as the eye could see there were undulating hills and streams. We were hooked. The sale went through without a hitch and we drove back to Germany. With the purchase of the house, a subtle change had taken place. Now there was no anxiety about retirement, we knew we had a home waiting to welcome us. The house in Ruislip was being let so the Pembrokeshire cottage became our retreat when we came home on leave.

For my last year before retirement I wanted a job with school holidays so that I could spend more time in Pembrokeshire in preparation for our return. As has happened so many times in my career, fate stepped in. The boarding school in Rinteln, about eight miles away, needed a nurse. I was overjoyed. To spend my last year in Germany doing a job that I loved. What could be better? My colleague at Prince Rupert School was Yvonne, the wife of the station padre. She was a joy to work with and became a great friend. I always say that I finished my career on a high. PRS was my favourite job ever. The atmosphere at the boarding house was always friendly. There was always something going on. For the younger pupils there was a drama group and they put on a show every year. The year I was there they had, 'Jungle Book.' Kay, the headmaster's wife organised the younger ones into a chorus. She found some concertina'd tubing from somewhere to make elephant trunks. The children paraded round the stage singing, 'the elephant dawn patrol.' One of the teachers found a bear costume and he played Balou the Bear. I will always remember it. The school had a pop group and there were frequent concerts. I often wonder what became of the lad who was the lead singer, he was a real performer. I can't remember his name though I have tried and tried.

There is always one pupil who stands out. At PRS, it was Alan. If there was mischief he was at the centre of it. They say some people are accident prone. Alan was. He came to sick bay having jumped off a wardrobe. I thought he may have fractured his wrist so I sent him to hospital for an X ray. He was duly plastered up and sent back. Two days later I spotted him in the schoolyard minus the plaster. I called him over and asked what had happened to it. "It was itching so I cut it off," he replied cheekily. I replaced it with a stiff strap on support and threatened him with all manner of penalties if he took this one off.

Every year there was a, 'no smoking day,' usually in March. Yvonne and I made posters and did all we could to publicise it. A competition was held between the schools to design a publicity pack so Yvonne and I got to work. We had a red, green, and amber theme.

Designing a life sized set of traffic lights out of cardboard, we used this to illustrate talks. Green was for a person who had never smoked, amber was someone who used to smoke but had stopped, and red was for smokers. We devised a lecture around this theme. We were thrilled to learn that our school had won the competition. We received a pack containing a T shirt, two baseball caps and numerous pens and key rings with the, 'No Smoking day,' logo on them. Yvonne and I wore the baseball caps around sick bay for the rest of the day. We then decided we had to do something with them rather than stash them away in a cupboard. We decided to have a competition among the pupils for the best, 'no smoking,' advert, with the T shirt as first prize and the two baseball caps for the runners up. The headmaster judged it and the winners were presented with their prizes in the morning assembly.

The headmaster's study was down the corridor from the sick bay, and I noticed that the same boy was standing outside the door more often than was usual. He wasn't one of the, 'Jack the lads,' that were always in trouble, normally he was quiet and polite. Although

I was reluctant to interfere, I felt I had to get to the bottom of this. I popped into the head's office and remarked on the number of times this lad was in trouble. The head told me that Jason was often sent to his office by the teachers because he was disruptive in class. I asked if he had always been like this and the head replied that, prior to the last year there hadn't been a problem with him. I happened to know, from my time in Herford medical centre, that Jason's mother had recently been diagnosed with a serious illness and was spending a lot of time in hospital. I struggled with my conscience. Do I break a confidence and discuss a patient, or do I tactfully explain that Jason was under a lot of strain and was acting it out in class. Without going into details, I told the headmaster what I thought might be the reason for Jason's behaviour. It wasn't a miracle transformation, but at least the headmaster knew the cause, and would deal with Jason accordingly. I had just one year at Prince Rupert School when John reached retirement age and we prepared to move back to the UK. The tenants had moved out of our house in Ruislip so we put it on the market and moved down to Wales. The housing market was buoyant at the time and it sold quickly. Back in Pembrokeshire we went to register with the local doctor's surgery. After the usual health questions he asked if we wanted to join the cricket club. They were having a social evening that weekend and he invited us to attend as his guests.

Chapter 14
Haverfordwest and Llangwm.

It appeared that there was a lively social scene for such a small village. In the summer there was a scarecrow competition. It was a farming community and most of the local farmers joined in the fun. Every other house had a scarecrow in their garden. They ranged from scary ones to animated ones that would squirt you with water when you walked past. This scarecrow competition became famous locally and attracted visitors from miles around. Also there was a lively arts and crafts scene. I had been dabbling with silk painting along with my other hobbies while in Germany so I had a supply of blank silk scarves and silk painting equipment. Finding myself with time on my hands for the first time in years, I threw myself wholeheartedly into this hobby. I had amassed a collection of about thirty painted scarves. Now what was I to do with them? At the cricket club dinner one of the ladies on our table invited me to join the local Women's Institute. My impression of the WI was similar, I suspect, to many other people who were not familiar with its workings. When the WI was mentioned it conjured up visions of righteous middle aged ladies peddling jam and singing Jerusalem.

I am not one for joining organisations, normally I even avoid coffee mornings. Call me unsociable, but that's just the way I am. Anyway, I had forgotten about the invitation when I received a phone call. It was the lady from the cricket club dinner. "Shall I pick you up about 7pm?" She asked. I was taken by surprise and had to think quickly. Then I remembered her invitation to the WI. There was no option but to accept her offer. This chance encounter opened up a whole new phase for me. The WI have frequent competitions and many openings for art and craft. This was just what I needed, an outlet for my frustrated creativity. The ladies proved to be a warm and welcoming crowd, and very soon I felt I was one of the gang. I joined the craft committee and found myself involved in projects that I would never have thought possible. My list of hobbies grew to include latex moulds for making concrete Celtic plaques and garden gnomes, large airbrushed posters as a backing for a millennium display, wood carving, making wooden mobiles of father Christmas and his reindeers and even poetry writing. There was a competition for a poem about Pembrokeshire so I put pen to paper. It didn't win but it went into our WI magazine.

John and I were on holiday in Greece when my mobile phone rang. It was the president of our WI. She told me that the committee had elected me as secretary in my absence. I was flabbergasted! She had no idea I was in Greece at the time. She said she had rung our home phone and got the answerphone, so rang the mobile number. I didn't know who was more surprised, me for being elected, or her, for finding out she was calling me in Greece. The way the WI worked was that if you were unable to do any committee work you could opt out, otherwise it was assumed you were available and willing. I always used to joke about how I was elected without my knowledge. Probably because nobody else wanted to do it. Being the secretary involved contacting the speakers for the monthly meetings and all the correspondence and thank you letters. It wasn't arduous and I learned a bit about organisation.

By that time Sara had moved from London and was working as publicity officer for St John's ambulance. She had a small house on the outskirts of Cardiff. I drove up one weekend for a girlie shopping trip. I was surprised to see a smart, well cut Christian Dior suit hanging behind her bedroom door, and was intrigued to know who the owner was. Not wanting to appear nosey, I waited a whole day before finally giving in and asking her. "I wondered when you would weaken." She laughed. Apparently, James was an engineer working in London. They had been going out for a month or so. Sara had had an eclectic taste in men, causing John and I some anxiety over the years. This one sounded reasonable. We were to meet him at my niece's wedding in three weeks time. That explained the suit behind the bedroom door.

Our son Jim was married to Lizzy, a lovely girl he had met while working at the BBC. They came down to Pembrokeshire for a week at Easter 1998. The usual chatter was going on around the dining table when Jim said. "Lizzy is having a baby." I wasn't really listening, but it suddenly dawned on me what he had said. "What did you just say?" I asked, not quite believing my ears. Jim repeated it and Lizzy had a broad smile on her face. I jumped up and enveloped them both in a big hug. We were overjoyed.

In due course Anna arrived, a tiny spiky haired bundle. We went to visit her at the hospital and there was Lizzy in tartan pyjamas, sitting cross legged on the bed, holding this tiny little girl. It was one of the proudest moments of my life. Driving back from the hospital we were overtaken by a car swerving in and out of the traffic dangerously. "That's some old grandad driving," said John. "So you're not an old grandad then," I replied. We suddenly realised that we were now officially Nanny and Grandad.

Rural life ambled along in Llangwm. A ploughing contest was advertised in the West Wales paper so we went along. Most of the local farmers were taking part. We saw old fashioned wooden ploughs drawn by magnificent shire horses. There were stalls selling hot potatoes and farmers fare. There was a lot of lively banter between the rival farmers. John stopped to talk to one of the farmers who was leading a big grey stallion. As they chatted John was rubbing the horse's nose. When he stopped the horse nudged him as if to say 'Hey, don't stop, I like it.' Every so often, while driving to Haverfordwest, the road would be blocked by a farmer driving his cows to another field. His old sheep dog would expertly herd the cows, and any calf that was tempted to stray was quickly brought into line. The dog would rush around directing the cows, while the farmer walked behind with his stick. The old dog would look at the farmer as if to say, 'Ignore him, I'm the one doing all the work'.

We soon settled in to the community but we found that our little holiday house had become too small for us, After moving from Germany and then from Ruislip we had accumulated a lot of furniture and belongings. When we first moved to Pembrokeshire I had admired a large self built house at the end of our lane but at the time we were only looking for a cottage. Miraculously, this house became available and so we sold the cottage and bought it. Now we had enough space to accommodate all the family for holidays and enough garage space for me to pursue my hobbies. Living in the country was a revelation to me. There was a badger set in the back garden and they would come out at night. We also had a fox. She came regularly to the

French windows, and, rightly or wrongly, we would put food out for her. I discovered that the neighbours did the same. She had a litter of four cubs and they would romp around like puppies. They would never come nearer than about ten yards. That seemed to be their safe distance. Two horses lived in the field over our fence and we fed them carrots. It was idyllic. A local farmer had a charolias bull. I have never seen such a big animal. He was magnificent. He was taller than me at the shoulder, with a massive head. The farmer said he was so placid you could fit a saddle on him. I wouldn't want to try.

Pembrokeshire is a mystical county with many ancient stones and monuments. There was Careg Samson, the subject of my painting, and Pentre Ifan, an ancient dolmen over a burial mound, also The Hanging Stone, to name but a few. How the prehistoric people managed to bring these massive stones inland and balance them on top of each other remains a mystery. It is widely supposed that the bluestones that make up Stonehenge came originally from the Preseli hills.

While we were in Wales, Mentor Preseli devised an ambitious plan to transport a sixteen ton bluestone from the Preseli hills to Stonehenge, some 240 miles, using the same methods that the Neolithic labourers had employed. The project was dogged with bad luck from the start. Having located a suitable stone in a farmer's field a team of volunteers built a huge sled and with the aid of a system of pulleys and ropes, loaded the stone on to it. They estimated that the volunteers, pulling the rope and levering from behind, would cover three miles a day. What they hadn't factored into this equation was the modern tarmac roads. The sled moved fairly smoothly over the rural tracks, but when they reached a tarmac road they discovered that it was practically impossible to pull it. This they solved by laying down green plastic sheeting. With the wet Welsh weather against them, they ploughed on, covering seventeen miles. With one day to go before they reached Milford Haven they discovered the sled was missing. This was a massive blow. Someone, obviously using heavy farm equipment, had stolen it. The stone was still there, but no longer any means of transporting it. After an extensive search, delaying the project still further, the sled was located hidden in a wood. The project was once again on track. The next obstacle was encountered when the volunteers reached the Bristol Channel. The stone was placed between two curraghs, long rowing boats. These were believed to be the means by which the original stones were transported. The rowers, with the stone slung between the boats, started their journey toward Milford Haven. They hadn't gone far when the stone began to slip from its harness and with a gurgle, slid beneath the waters of the Haven. Devastation all round. All was not lost. Assisted by divers, all volunteers, the stone was retrieved some eleven days later. The project was refloated. The final deathknell came when the original insurers withdrew their support. It was impossible to carry on such a hazardous project without insurance cover and, reluctantly it was abandoned. The stone, after lying on the quay in Milford Haven for some months, was eventually transported to the National Botanical Gardens of Wales, quite near to Pembrokeshire.

Soon after this Sara came down to Llangwm sporting an engagement ring. This was the beginning of months of frantic activity. Now there was a wedding to arrange. They had decided to get married at Castell Coch - The Red castle - a medieval type castle near Caerphilly. It was known locally as the fairy castle and was in a picturesque setting on a hill surrounded by trees. The turrets of the castle could be seen from the road, and when the mist was down it looked as if it was floating in the air. It was rebuilt in Victorian times over the ruins of a twelfth century castle on the instructions of the Marquis of Bute. He was one of the richest men in Wales due to the vast mineral wealth of iron and coal.

The logistics were somewhat complicated due to the fact that Sara chose a dressmaker who lived more than one hundred miles from Cardiff. This involved many trips down to the wilds of West Wales for the fittings. Her three bridesmaids also had dresses designed by Sara, and made by the same dressmaker. Two of these bridesmaids lived in London, so there was a lot of organising involved. This was left to me as I lived nearest to the seamstress. Also, there was the question of wedding favours. Sara wanted miniature Welsh love spoons tied with pink ribbon. We managed to locate a bulk supply of love spoons, but at midnight on the night before the wedding I was frantically tying on a hundred bows of pink ribbon. The day of the wedding dawned fine and sunny. Everything had come together and the weeks of planning and calming Sara down were all worthwhile. She looked beautiful. I know all brides look beautiful on their wedding day, but she really did. The dress was a resounding success. A white and gold bodice and a midnight blue shot silk skirt with a long train. It was quite an unusual dress, but then, Sara is quite an unusual girl. The venue for the reception was decked out with purple and silver balloons. We were serenaded throughout the meal by a harpist playing a massive golden harp accompanied by a flautist. The honeymoon couple flew off to Cyprus and John and I sat back and relaxed for the first time since the engagement was announced. It had been worth all the effort.

Meanwhile a recession had hit Wales, along with the rest of the UK. Our little post office had closed and soon after, the local shop ceased to trade. The housing market stagnated and for the next three years more and more shops in Haverfordwest had to close down. Sara's husband, James was also affected by the turndown. The firm he worked for was forced to lay off a large part of the workforce. Rather than wait for the axe to fall, he volunteered to pioneer a new venture in France. They both moved to France and set up home in a rented house. Sara got a job teaching English and in her spare time attempted to establish herself as a potter. The arts scene in France was accommodating and soon she had made friends among the artistic community. James moved to a permanent job, and gradually they became more fluent in French. Now it was time to decide whether to stay in France permanently. As Sara had travelled most of her life it was no big decision for her. They started house hunting.

We had taken several trips to France while Sara and James were settling in. At the time we had a camper van and would tour the vineyards and the battle fields of the Somme. We visited the Menin gate in Belgium, a memorial to the British and Commonwealth soldiers who had lost their lives in the great war at Ypres. We also visited the pristine military cemeteries at Abbeville, Bayeux and Loos. The French have cause to remember the war, and they kept the graves in immaculate condition.

Sara had two cats and she left them with us while they moved to France. When they were settled, we loaded the cats into the camper van and proceeded through the channel tunnel with both of them sitting proudly on the dashboard. We had taken them to the vets to be microchipped and to get their pet passports ready for the journey. We wondered what 'miaou' was in French.

With Sara and James in France, and Jim and Lizzy in Nottingham we began to feel isolated in Pembrokeshire. The nearest big town was Carmarthen, some fifty miles each way. With the local shop and the post office closed we began to wonder if we really were ready to settle down permanently. The answer was a resounding 'no'.

Chapter 15

A French Idyll.

After some months of deliberating and weighing up the pro's and cons of uprooting ourselves again, we made the big decision. There was no question of selling up in UK. We were Brits. Wherever we had travelled in the world, UK was home. So it was that we embarked on a year long search for just the right house in France. It wasn't our plan to live right next door to Sara, we thought it was better to give them some space. We didn't want to be the inlaws from hell. The search for a house began in the Cognac region. There seemed to be an endless supply of empty properties. The problem was that ninety percent of them were ruins. There was no shortage of land and we were shown ramshackle farmhouses with acres of land but the living accommodation was falling down. This was partly due to the French laws. In French law a property must be divided between all the surviving children in equal shares. France, being a mainly catholic country, they tended to have large families. Often the siblings could not agree on how to manage the property. Some were anxious to sell up, but others would want to keep it or even live in it. Consequently, while this dispute continued the property would fall into disrepair. These fueds would fester on until the next generation. None if them could agree on who would pay for the necessary repairs. We saw some horrendous houses before moving our search to Brittany where the problems were much the same.

Our estate agent, Gaston, was a dour Frenchman. There appeared to be two types of estate agent. One was charming, garrulous, devastatingly handsome and slightly flirtatious. The other kind was taciturn and dour. Of the three properties we were shown, one was open on to a main road with no pavement. The rooms were large with high ceilings. Long narrow windows with small panes of glass dominated the room. Faded flowering wallpaper covered the walls and, surprisingly, the doors. There was a drainy smell. The owners, an old couple, were anxious to sell up and move to one of the newly built modern houses that were springing up everywhere. We didn't want modern, we wanted old fashioned and charming.

Unfortunately, old fashioned and charming came with a lot of work. The second house was a nightmare. Rusting farm machinery lay haphazardly around the overgrown garden. A large sewage pipe stretched diagonally across the living room wall. We wouldn't have believed it possible if we hadn't seen it with our own eyes. The bathroom walls were covered in mould and the bath looked as if it had been used for anything but bathing. I won't mention the toilet, it still makes me shudder. We set out for the third house, not holding out much hope. Suddenly Gaston looked at his watch. "It is the hour." He said, turning the car and heading for home. Lunch hour is sacrosanct in France. Nothing, but *nothing*, is allowed to interfere with lunch. Based on that days experience we decided to forego the third visit. A story is told that in the second world war, British clandestine forces were parachuted into a resistance stronghold near to enemy territory. Their mission was to locate the resistance cell, deliver vital plans and disappear quickly. The Frenchmen insisted in shaking hands all round and sitting them down for lunch.

Another estate agency near Beaumont appeared more promising. It was June and the fields were red with acres and acres of poppies. This time our agent, Dominic, was one of the first category, charming and flirtatious. He too, had three properties on his books. The first one he showed us was a stunningly beautiful old house. Massive oak beams and a gigantic stone fireplace dominated the room. Upstairs the bedrooms were in the process of renovation. The house was on three storeys and the third storey was being converted into a separate flat. There was a gap between the two upper storeys with no barrier and a six foot drop to the floor below. We couldn't see how this could be rectified without major structural work. Reluctantly we put it on our 'reject' list. The second property was promising. It even had a swimming pool. In a reasonable state of repair, it was in the centre of a village. We were quite taken with it until we realised it backed on to an undertakers. It had just a dividing wall between the living room and a funeral parlour. We drove for another four or five miles, deeper into the countryside until we came to an isolated farmhouse. There were vineyards surrounding it and walnut trees lined the walk to a wrought iron gate. Dominic strode proudly up to the gate. He sensed that we were almost ready to compromise and choose a house that, although it wasn't our dream house, it would meet most of our needs. Fishing in his pocket, he withdrew a large bunch of keys. The first one didn't fit the lock. With a Gallic shrug, he tried another one. After trying all ten of the keys on his bunch he reluctantly conceded that the lock must have been changed. The lock, like the gates, was ancient and rusty. It certainly hadn't been changed recently. Once again we drove back as it was lunchtime.

France in 2000 was like stepping back in time fifty years. The pace of life was much slower than in UK, slower even, than in Pembrokeshire. Apart from the big towns, one could drive for miles on the motorway and see only a handful of cars. Part of the reason for this is that the French motorways have tolls. The French system is, in a way, fairer as they don't pay road tax, just insurance. This means that French drivers only pay when they want to use the motorway. Having said that, it can work out quite expensive for long journeys. Even on the Route Nationale, one may drive through villages and not see a soul. It's as if there has been an alien invasion and all the inhabitants have been spirited away. The health and safety laws seem non existent. We passed labourers using stone cutting equipment on a building site. The air was thick with cement dust but there wasn't a mask or a pair of goggles in sight. Every other workman was smoking. The wooden scaffolding on some of the buildings looked precarious, to say the least.

Our search took us to Chinon, a prolific wine growing region. It had a magnificent castle set on a hill overlooking the town and was divided by the river Vienne. A long shopping street stretched from one side of the town to the other with numerous little roads leading to specialist boutiques and art galleries. I could have lingered there all day. Three main estate agents vied for customers in the main street. Looking in their windows we saw properties very similar to what we had been shown before Our enthusiasm began to wane. Was every property in France going to be so decrepit that it would take us half a lifetime to renovate. We were due to go back to UK the following week and we had hoped to find somewhere nice in France this time.

We had now been searching for a year. There was one more estate agency in Chinon. We had seen this one several times but it appeared to be a one man operation and not as high profile as the others. We hadn't bothered to look inside. While taking a break and sipping thick dark coffee at a roadside cafe, John suggested that we have a look at this one. "We go back next week, we have nothing to lose," he said. "Ever the optimist." I replied with as much sarcasm as humour. By this time my feet were aching and I had had enough. The little shop was cramped inside with a large counter dominating the reception area. The folders of properties were looking dog eared and neglected. Eventually Mr Quincaneau came out from behind the counter. He was a fussy little man with sparse grey hair and wire rimmed glasses. He appeared nervous, his speech and movements were jerky, not a man to put you at your ease. We were invited to sit down and he asked us what exactly we were looking for. This was a surprise, as all the other estate agents had just seemed to guess what we wanted because we were British. No one had asked us to be specific. It seemed to us that their objective had been to offload houses rather than to address the client's special requirements. Mr Quincaneau even had a check list. As we enunciated exactly what we were looking for the picture became clearer in our minds. The previous year of searching had appeared tedious at times, but it had done much to narrow down our view of what we wanted. Basically, we wanted an old house with charm but not in need of too much expensive work. "So," said our man. "You want a renovated property, do you want land?" "Not so much that we can't maintain it." We replied. "This property, must it be in a village or do you want ..." He hesitated. He was looking for the right word. "Solitude." We didn't mind, by this time, if he had offered the right house on the moon we would have taken it. "I would like to show you three properties," he said, now sounding much more businesslike. This was a revelation. Any one of the three properties would have suited us. The first one was just outside Chinon. Surrounded by vineyards, it was approached down a leafy but slightly rutted track. An imposing facade in French Manor House style stopped us in our tracks. This was a mansion. The owner and his wife came out to meet us. We were offered wine from the vineyard and started on a tour of the house. It had been tastefully renovated in keeping with the original style. The living room was as big as a ballroom, with large oak beams and high windows. The quarry tiled floor added charm and the colourful rugs scattered around added warmth. Two massive bedrooms led off to a blue tiled bathroom. A modern shower cubicle with a power shower stood on one side while a white porcelain free standing bath with claw feet occupied the rest of the room.

The next house was about fifteen miles in the other direction. That, too, was newly renovated. A totally different style of house, it was a *longere*. a French farmhouse all on one storey, stretched out with all the buildings on one level. The roofspace had been converted into two bedrooms with the study, bathroom and living area at ground level. The grounds were extensive, with a smaller cottage and stables as part of the deal. There was a barn attached to the side of the house, which had been made into a small workshop. The garden was a riot of colour. There was wisteria and hollyhocks, as well as what appeared to be acres of grapevines. Rows of beans stood to attention like sentinels. We began to feel excited.

It was the third house that really got our attention. We drove deeper into the countryside, through deserted villages, passing acres of ever present vineyards and fields with herds of brown cows. Every so often we would pass a monument to a resistance fighter, bringing to mind the horrors that the French people had endured in their own country. "Nous sommes arrivez," proclaimed Mr Quincaneau. We have arrived. The house was in the centre of a village, Neuilly le Brignon. A massive studded oak door set in a wall decorated with pargetted plasterwork led into a courtyard with an enclosed garden. A well with a bucket on a chain stood in a corner and behind it was a tiled picnic area with a wooden sign - 'Le Buffet.' To the left of that was a large building with a dirt floor, wooden beams and a wooden structure with a trench below it. Mr Quincaneau said it was for hay to feed the cows. At one time this had been a working farmhouse. The room would be ideal for a studio to house my ever growing collection of tools and art materials. I could also use my airbrush without worrying about spraying the walls and furniture. We were half convinced before we even set foot inside the house.

Mr Quincaneau unlocked the door to the main living room. We gasped! It was beautiful. High ceilings, oak beams and an old iron fireplace. Rough stone walls with alcoves high up for ornaments, stone tiled floors and a gigantic wooden light fitting with nine electric candles. A staircase in the corner led up to the bathroom with built in cupboards, a white bath and shower. The bathroom was almost as big as the living room. Another short flight of steps led up to a study, two large bedrooms and another bedroom on a slightly higher level. Every bedroom had fitted wardrobes and everything was in immaculate condition. The price, by English standards, was ridiculously low. We got back to the hotel and weighed up all three properties. By this time our minds were made up. The third house had the advantage of being in a village with a little shop and it was easily accessible by road. Apart from that, the walled garden afforded privacy and the workshop was ideal. We went back and slept on it, but the decision was already made.

First thing next morning we contacted Mr Quincaneau. He set the wheels in motion to complete the sale. John took photographs and drove to Le Mans to tell Sara and James, who couldn't wait to drive down and see it. Two months later the formalities were completed and we met in the notaire's office to sign the paperwork

Here we go again, another move. This time it's our choice and we are calling the shots. The last two months were spent in arranging for our house in Pembrokeshire to be let on a short lease and contacting furniture removal firms. At last we were ready for the move. The long drive to France was lightened by the fact that we were finally moving into our house, the one that we had spent a year searching for. The delivery van met us at the appointed time. The driver looked as if he had spent the night in his cab, bleary eyed and unshaven.

One of the new neighbours wandered over and started a conversation in French. I was taken aback! I thought my schoolgirl French was reasonably good but I couldn't understand a word he said. From his expression, the way he kissed me on both cheeks and shook John's hand, I gathered that he was welcoming us to the village. The next few days heralded a procession of local people from the village. It was all very informal. We were introduced to the mayor, who was also the local shopkeeper. As the weather was warm I had the window open on to the street. Pierre, the man next door, popped his head in through and started a conversation. I struggled to understand him when he threw his hands up in the air and disappeared. I was quite upset until twenty minutes later he reappeared with a lady, also leaning in through the window. She was the local schoolmistress and spoke some English.

As the weeks went on we managed to decipher the local dialect. It was French, of course, but not the French I had been taught more than forty years ago. It was a steep learning curve. We were invited to the community centre for a lunch. Practically everyone in the village was there. It started with aperitifs and bread rolls, presumably to mop up the alcohol. Everyone then milled around for half an hour, then we all piled in to a room with long trestle tables decorated with flowers and miniature tricolours. The first course was a fish concoction served with copious amounts of white wine. There were speeches and general hubbub then there was what I can only describe as a kind of vol au vent, or pasty with red wine. An interval of half an hour, then came the main course, Chicken in white wine with vegetables. More wine, this time a choice of white or red. More chatter, then came the cheese. A plate with goat's cheese produced from the farm up the road, camembert and pont l'eveque, a pungent cheese that is popular with the French although you could smell it a mile away. This was served with salad and, of course, more wine. Another pause, then a sorbet with champagne. Last of all, a creme caramel and more champagne. The mayor came round finally with bottles of brandy or peach liqueur. By then it was getting on for five thirty. We had been at lunch for five hours. This, apparently, was normal. There was a lunch every few months whether it was for armistice day, Saints day or the annual football club do.

The village shops sold French baguettes and most mornings I would stroll up for my morning loaf. The trouble was, it was not a straightforward journey. It seemed that everyone was out on the street and I would have to shake hands or kiss everyone I met. A simple nod or 'Bonjour' wouldn't do, it had to be a kiss. This is the custom in France, but to a fairly reserved Brit, it took a lot of getting used to. And again, I never knew whether it was two or four kisses.

The house next door was another ancient building in the process of being modernised. Yvette and Christian, the owners, were retiling the roof. The three workmen they employed had the same disregard for health and safety as most of their colleagues. The three hundred year old slates were thrown haphazardly from the roof into a skip. Sometimes they landed, sometimes they did not. I picked up one or two from our garden and my creative urges kicked in. The slate was covered in lichen and was a smoky blue colour. It just spoke to me. Taking it into my workshop I traced a dragon from a Celtic design in one of my books and proceeded to engrave it with a stone drill. I bored two holes and threaded them with silver cord, carved a Celtic border around the edges, and gave it to Yvette. She was thrilled, and promptly hung it up on her wall

Our courtyard played host to a variety of wildlife, not all of them welcome. Stepping over the threshold into my workshop, I bent to pick up what I thought was a piece of black and grey string. It moved. It was a baby adder. There were grass snakes, a bat that looked exactly like a mouse with wings, two rats, caterpillars, a stag beetle, crickets, hundreds of little black and red beetles that appeared every spring and disappeared in the autumn. Coming home from a weekend away we heard a strange humming noise in the living room. We traced it to the hearth and discovered a swarm of bees in the chimney. Fortunately the fireplace had a glass door which we kept closed unless there was a log fire. Another time we had to call in the pest controller to get rid of hornets in the kitchen chimney.

The river Brignon ran through the village and it regularly flooded when there was heavy rain. It always flooded over the play park on the opposite side of the road. The water receded as quickly as it had appeared, and by the next morning everything was back to normal. We discovered after living in the house for a few months, that in the 1940's German occupation our house had been the headquarters, or the commandateria, of the occupying forces. Madame Hainault, a neighbour, tells the story of when she was a teenager. None of the French villagers were allowed a radio so Madame Hainault and her friends used to go over to the German Headquarters and listen to dance music on the soldier's radio. Not everyone in occupied France was SS or a Nazi.

Our village, Neuilly le Brignon was renamed round about 1798, when before the upheaval of the storming of the Bastille in 1798 and the subsequent French revolution, it had been called Neuilly le Noble. Following the revolution, when all signs of the aristocracy were being obliterated, it became known a Neuilly le Brignon, as it still is today. Many French villages were renamed to reflect the new order after execution of Louis XV1 in 1793. 'The Terror', from 1793 to 1794 when fifty to sixty people daily were summarily executed at any one time, saw the mass evacuation and escape of many aristocrats to neighbouring European countries.

We discovered, after moving into the house, that we had also purchased a plot of land. Mr Quincaneau had omitted to tell us about this. It wasn't until we came to sign the deeds, that it came to light. Jean Paul, a farmer had had an agreement with the previous owners, whereby he farmed the plot of land in exchange for occasional baskets of fruit and vegetables. So it was that, every season there would be a knock on the door, and Jean Paul would be standing there with a basket of aubergines, tomatoes, plums and whatever else happened to be growing on our land at the time. This arrangement suited us as neither John or I had any aptitude for farming. Jean Paul would be invited in and the whisky bottle would be brought out. It was a satisfactory arrangement all round.

After seven years of living partly in France and partly in Wales we began to think about where we wanted to settle permanently. France, with her fields of sunflowers in the autumn and poppies in the spring was beautiful, and her health service was second to none, but it was a long drive every few months. We finally decided that our French idyll was over and tentatively enquired about selling up. The estate agent in Descarte was a young, dynamic woman, quite different from the dozy agents we had encountered previously. She came to view the house and persuaded us to put it on the market. Our house in Pembrokeshire had been on the market for three years with no interest whatsoever, so we were quite unprepared for what happened next. Within a week we had a buyer. It was a total shock. With hindsight, this galvanised our plans, as we would probably have dithered for a few more years. We began the difficult business of deciding what furniture to take back to UK. We had accumulated a lot of baggage after seven years in France

One small surprise awaited us. When we came to move our furniture out, and the house was clear, we discovered a hollow patch under the floor tiles in the living room. There was obviously a cellar or something that had been tiled over during the many renovations that the house had undergone over the centuries. Of course, we couldn't go lifting the floor up to see what was underneath. Jean Paul's wife suggested an escape tunnel from the eighteenth century, and, more darkly, Jean Paul suggested it might be a body. In a way I was glad that we hadn't discovered it while we were living there. Eventually we arrived back in Pembrokeshire just as the housing market was turning. Within a month our house, which had been on the market for three years, suddenly had three bidders competing for a sale. If we weren't careful we would be homeless.

Suddenly we found ourselves frantically searching for somewhere to live. This was an important decision because it was likely to be our last house. It had to be right. We had moved so many times over the years that we had a good idea of the kind of place we wanted. We now had four grandchildren and it would be nice to see them growing up. Nottingham seemed central to most places and it was where our son and his wife lived. After looking at the many houses available we settled on a smaller four bedroomed house in a village, just fifteen minutes away from the family. There was a regular bus service into Nottingham city centre every fifteen minutes. From there we could go on to Derby, Grantham, Leicester and Newark. Even Chesterfield was only an hour and a half away. As we both had bus passes we seldom even needed to use the car.

At last, after forty years of travelling I was finally where I wanted to be. We had had a life full of adventure and we hadn't finished yet. My next challenge was nothing to do with blue lights and ambulances. Now I had to master the intricacies of using a computer. Looking back over a life spent following the drum, I wouldn't change a thing.

Also by Maud Harris.

Three Years in Starch.

Three Years in Starch is the story of general nurse training in a large teaching hospital in the West Country from late 1950's to early 1960's.Read about night duty on the haunted ward, the man on the balcony with a gun, the day sisters muslin cap fell in the bathwater. The policeman who accused us of stealing his pint of milk and much more, both hilarious and poignant.

Sarah Sunshine and the elves.

A children's book for ages 5 to 7 with short, easily readable chapters. Sarah Sunshine knew there were elves, she just didn't know where to find them. Read about her adventures as she seeks them out, culminating in being made an honorary elf.

The Quota.

Teenage/ young adult thriller. The story of a
damaged young man who collects dolls - human dolls.
His quota is four. Read what happens when he has
collected all four. Can DI Livingstone stop him in
time?

Amazon B009QL4IIE

Short Stories and Poems.
A collection of flash fiction tales ranging from the
snowy steppes of Russia, through occupied France,
London, Scotland, America and Switzerland. Between
the covers can be found historical fiction, crime,
romance, science fiction, space travel and a small
section of poetry. Each story is complete in itself and
will take the reader on a journey.
Amazon B01181MMIC

www.ingramcontent.com/pod-product-compliance
Lightning Source LLC
Chambersburg PA
CBHW021422170526
45164CB00001B/53